MEDICAL MANAGEMENT OF
PREGNANCY
COMPLICATED
BY DIABETES

SIXTH EDITION

Edited by
Erika Werner, MD

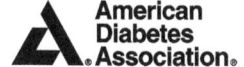

American
Diabetes
Association.

Associate Publisher, Books, Abe Ogden; *Director, Book Operations*, Victor Van Beuren; *Managing Editor, Books*, John Clark; *Associate Director, Book Marketing*, Annette Reape; *Acquisitions Editor*, Jaclyn Konich; *Senior Manager, Book Editing*, Lauren Wilson; *Composition*, Cenveo Publisher Services; *Cover Design*, American Diabetes Association; *Printer*, Lightning Source®.

Printed in the United States of America
1 3 5 7 9 10 8 6 4 2

The suggestions and information contained in this publication are generally consistent with the *Standards of Medical Care in Diabetes* and other policies of the American Diabetes Association, but they do not represent the policy or position of the Association or any of its boards or committees. Reasonable steps have been taken to ensure the accuracy of the information presented. However, the American Diabetes Association cannot ensure the safety or efficacy of any product or service described in this publication. Individuals are advised to consult a physician or other appropriate health care professional before undertaking any diet or exercise program or taking any medication referred to in this publication. Professionals must use and apply their own professional judgment, experience, and training and should not rely solely on the information contained in this publication before prescribing any diet, exercise, or medication. The American Diabetes Association—its officers, directors, employees, volunteers, and members—assumes no responsibility or liability for personal or other injury, loss, or damage that may result from the suggestions or information in this publication.

Matt Petersen conducted the internal review of this book to ensure that it meets American Diabetes Association guidelines.

∞ The paper in this publication meets the requirements of the ANSI Standard Z39.48-1992 (permanence of paper).

ADA titles may be purchased for business or promotional use or for special sales. To purchase more than 50 copies of this book at a discount, or for custom editions of this book with your logo, contact the American Diabetes Association at the address below or at booksales@diabetes.org.

American Diabetes Association
2451 Crystal Drive, Suite 900
Arlington, VA 22202

DOI: 10.2337/9781580406987

Library of Congress Cataloging-in-Publication Data
Names: Werner, Erika, editor. | American Diabetes Association.
Title: Medical management of pregnancy complicated by diabetes / [edited by] Erika Werner.
Description: 6th edition. | Arlington : American Diabetes Association, [2019] | Includes bibliographical references and index.
Identifiers: LCCN 2018050557 | ISBN 9781580406987 (softcover : alk. paper)
Subjects: | MESH: Pregnancy in Diabetics–therapy | Diabetes, Gestational–therapy | Diabetes Mellitus | Pregnancy Outcome
Classification: LCC RG580.D5 | NLM WQ 248 | DDC 618.3–dc23 LC record available ps://lccn.loc.gov/2018050557

Contents

Foreword

This sixth edition is intended to provide updated guidance on the care of pregnant women with preexisting diabetes, including both types 1 and type 2 diabetes, as well as women with gestational diabetes mellitus. The care of pregnant women with diabetes and gestational diabetes mellitus requires a committed healthcare team and considerable resources. It is our hope that the information in this book will be helpful in enabling the various healthcare professionals who make up that team to have access to practical advice and carry out their mission. Each of the contributors is engaged actively in optimizing the care of pregnant women with diabetes either through clinical care or research. Although there are many reasonable approaches to providing that care, we have outlined herein those that we find to be most effective.

Acknowledgments

The last edition of this book was edited by Dr. Donald Coustan, a gifted clinician, educator, and researcher. Dr. Coustan has mentored many of us who now care for women with diabetes in pregnancy. His work has forever changed diabetes-in-pregnancy care and inspired the next generation of diabetes-in-pregnancy leaders. Although we have updated this edition, the fifth edition was beyond thorough, and as such, we used it as the foundation for most of what is included here. Therefore, we would like to acknowledge the important contributions of the many health professionals who contributed to previous editions of this book.

Susan Biastre, RD, LDN, CDE

Richard M. Cowett, MD

Julie M. Daley, RN, MS, CDE

Stephanie Dunbar, MPH, RD

Carol J. Homko, RN, PhD, CDE

Donna Jornsay, RN, BSN, CPNP, MSS, ACSW

Sue Kirkman, MD

John L. Kitzmiller, MD

Siri Kjos, MD, MSEd

Abbot R. Laptook, MD

Lisa Marasco, MA, IBCLC, FILCA

Noreen Hall Papatheodorou, MSS, ACSW

Anne M. Patterson, RD, MPH

List of New Contributors

Nansi S. Boghossian, PhD, MPH
Assistant Professor
Arnold School of Public Health of
    University of South Carolina
Department of Epidemiology and
    Biostatistics
Columbia, SC

Ebony Boyce Carter, MD, MPH
Assistant Professor
Washington University School of
    Medicine
Department of Obstetrics and
    Gynecology
St. Louis, MO

Erin Cleary, MD
Assistant Professor
Warren Alpert Medical School of
    Brown University
Obstetrics and Gynecology
Women and Infants Hospital of
    Rhode Island
Providence, RI

Maureen Hamel, MD
Assistant Professor
University of Pittsburgh
Division of Maternal Fetal Medicine
Pittsburgh, PA

Christina Han, MD
Associate Professor
University of California, Los Angeles
Obstetrics and Gynecology
Center for Fetal Medicine and
    Women's Ultrasound
Los Angeles, CA

Lorie Harper, MD, MSCI
Associate Professor
University of Alabama at Birmingham
Division of Maternal-Fetal Medicine
Birmingham, AL

Teri L. Hernandez, PhD, RN
Associate Professor of Medicine and
    Nursing
University of Colorado, Anschutz
    Medical Campus
Department of Medicine, Division of
    Endocrinology, Metabolism, and
    Diabetes
Denver, CO

Pre- and Interpregnancy Counseling, Assessment, and Management

Highlights
Pre- and Interpregnancy Counseling, Assessment, and Management

■ With proper counseling and management by the healthcare team, the outcome of most pregnancies complicated by diabetes can approach that of the general population.

■ General guidelines for prepregnancy counseling and management of women with preexisting diabetes are as follows:

- Ensure that pregnancy is planned; counsel the woman about contraception methods and their expected efficacy and failure rates.
- Clearly identify for the woman and her partner the risks of congenital anomalies and spontaneous abortions, and their relation to A1C leading up to conception.
- Achieve optimum control of blood glucose levels before conception. Ideally, A1C should be normal (6%) or near normal before discontinuing contraception.
- Provide realistic information about chronic complications of type 1 diabetes (T1D) and type 2 diabetes (T2D), their potential impact on pregnancy and childbearing, and the effect of pregnancy on chronic complications.

- Assess the woman's baseline health status, paying special attention to retinopathy, nephropathy, hypertension, neuropathy, and ischemic heart disease.
- Identify any gynecologic abnormalities before conception, and treat infertility as early as possible in view of the risk to pregnancy associated with increasing duration of diabetes and advancing maternal age.
- Provide genetic counseling, including the risks of advanced maternal age, if applicable.
- Provide realistic information about additional medical costs associated with a pregnancy complicated by diabetes, such as extra office visits, possible hospitalization, special tests, and possible intensive neonatal care.
- Encourage good general principles of health, nutrition, and hygiene, including cessation of smoking and alcohol consumption.
- Prescribe a prenatal vitamin with folate as part of the preconception treatment plan and review all other medications, making changes if teratogenic effects are possible.

- Identify any problems requiring psychosocial consultation.
- Once the decision is made to attempt pregnancy, provide appropriate optimism that careful glycemic control and meticulous obstetric care result in an excellent outcome in the vast majority of patients.
- Diagnose pregnancy as early as possible and document estimated due date.

■ Interpregnancy counseling and management of women with previous gestational diabetes mellitus should include the following:
- Testing for diabetes or prediabetes, measuring glucose levels, and assessing the need for treatment if diabetes or prediabetes is found.
- Evaluating weight status and advising weight reduction, if appropriate.
- Reviewing the risk of gestational diabetes mellitus in future pregnancy (~50% risk) and of T2D (up to 70% lifetime risk).
- Advising careful family planning with use of effective contraception until pregnancy is desired.

Pre- and Interpregnancy Counseling, Assessment, and Management

PREEXISTING DIABETES

Women with preexisting diabetes (type 1 diabetes [T1D] or type 2 diabetes [T2D]) who desire pregnancy present a broad array of challenging problems for the healthcare team. In the pre-insulin era, maternal mortality was as high as 44%, and perinatal mortality was 60% (Hare and White 1977). Children with true T1D, however, seldom lived to childbearing ages. After the discovery of insulin, maternal and fetal or neonatal survival improved dramatically. During the past five decades, advances in the care of the individual with diabetes in general, as well as advances in fetal surveillance and neonatal care, have continued to improve outcomes in most diabetic pregnancies to near that of the general population (Diabetes Control and Complications Trial Research Group 1996). The most common maternal (Table 1.1) and fetal or neonatal (Table 1.2) complications have decreased dramatically.

Table 1.1 — Examples of Maternal Complications in Diabetic Pregnancy

- Hypoglycemia, ketoacidosis
- Pregnancy-induced hypertension and preeclampsia
- Pyelonephritis, other infections
- Polyhydramnios
- Preterm labor
- Worsening of chronic complications—retinopathy, nephropathy, neuropathy, cardiac disease
- Delivery complications (cesarean, third- and fourth-degree lacerations)

Table 1.2—Examples of Potential Perinatal Morbidity or Mortality in Infants of Mothers with Diabetes

- Asphyxia
- Birth injury
- Cardiac hypertrophy and heart failure
- Congenital anomalies
- Erythremia (increased red blood cells) and hyperviscosity
- Hyperbilirubinemia
- Hypocalcemia
- Hypoglycemia
- Hypomagnesemia
- Intrauterine growth restriction
- Macrosomia
- Neurological instability; irritability
- Organomegaly
- Respiratory distress syndrome
- Stillbirth

Morbidity and mortality associated with major congenital anomalies and spontaneous abortion (SAB) are of major concern in preexisting T1D and T2D. The magnitude of both appears to be related to metabolic control. The true prevalence of SAB pregnancies is not known, but it has been reported to be as high as 30–60%, depending on the degree of hyperglycemia at the time of conception, which is double that of the general population (Miodovnik et al. 1984). The increased risk of congenital anomalies among women with T1D ranges from 6%–12%, a two- to fivefold increase over the 2–3% incidence observed in the general population (Kitzmiller et al. 1978, Reece et al. 1988, Bell et al. 2012). This increased risk of congenital anomalies accounts for ~40% of the perinatal loss in T1D (Reece and Hobbins 1986). The combined risk of congenital anomalies and SAB in poorly controlled diabetes in early pregnancy can approach 65% (Greene 1993). In a nationwide prospective study, which included first-trimester questionnaires filled out by all pregnant women with T1D in the Netherlands over a 1-year interval, congenital malformations occurred in 4.2% of self-reported planned pregnancies but in 12.2% of unplanned pregnancies (Evers et al. 2004). Congenital malformations also increased when the mother has T2D (Macintosh et al. 2006) or obesity (Watkins et al. 2003). It is speculated that the relationship between obesity and anomalies is related to undiagnosed T2D; with an anticipated increased prevalence of undiagnosed T2D, a parallel increase in congenital anomalies also can be expected (Zabihi and Loeken 2010).

The types of congenital anomalies observed in diabetes are varied (Table 1.3). Most are of cardiac, neural tube, or skeletal origin; they are more commonly multiple, more severe, and more often fatal than those found in the general population.

Table 1.3—Congenital Anomaly Rates in Pregnancies of Women with and without Preexisting Diabetes per 1,000 Singleton Pregnancies and Relative Risk (95% Confidence Interval [CI])

Anomalies	Pregnancies with Diabetes		Pregnancies without Diabetes		Relative Risk (95% CI)
	n	Rate (95% CI)	n	Rate (95% CI)	
Nervous System	16	9.5 (5.4, 15.4)	769	1.9 (1.8, 2.1)	5 (3.0, 8.1)
Neural Tube Defects	10	6 (2.9, 10.9)	443	1.1 (1.0, 1.2)	5.4 (2.9, 10.1)
Cardiovascular System	44	26.2 (19.1, 35.1)	2,919	7.3 (7.0, 7.6)	3.6 (2.7, 4.8)
Ventricular Septal Defect	21	12.5 (7.8, 19.1)	1,285	3 (3.0, 3.4)	3.9 (2.6, 6.0)
Digestive System	10	6 (2.9, 10.9)	421	1.05 (0.95, 1.15)	5.7 (3.0, 10.6)
Urinary	12	7.2 (3.7, 12.5)	974	2.4 (2.3, 2.6)	2.9 (1.7, 5.2)
Musculoskeletal	3	1.8 (0.4, 5.2)	55	0.14 (0.1, 0.2)	13 (4.1, 41.5)
Syndrome (monogenic or unknown)	11	6.6 (3.2, 11.7)	439	1.1 (1.0, 1.2)	6 (3.1, 10.9)

Source: Adapted from Bell et al. (2012).

The etiology of the increased prevalence of congenital anomalies in diabetes has been the subject of intense research. In an experimental setting, hyperglycemia and other metabolic abnormalities are teratogenic, singly or in combination (Kalter and Warkany 1983, Freinkel et al. 1984, Reece and Hobbins 1986, Reece et al. 1988, Sadler et al. 1989). More recently, studies have demonstrated that biochemical disturbances and oxidative stress influence altered expression of essential developmental control genes; the timing of such environments may explain the unpredictable number or pattern of specific anomalies in any one fetus (Zabihi and Loeken 2010). Fetal organogenesis is largely complete by 9 weeks after the last menstrual period (7 weeks postconception) (Mills et al. 1979). Poorly controlled diabetes during the early weeks of pregnancy, in many cases before a woman even knows that she has conceived, significantly increases the risk of a first-trimester SAB or delivering an infant with a major anomaly (Greene et al. 1989).

The glycosylated hemoglobin or A1C, which expresses an average of the circulating glucose for the 2–3 months before its measurement, has become a useful tool in assessing a woman's metabolic control early in pregnancy, during the critical period of organogenesis. Several studies have shown a definite association between A1C levels in early pregnancy (<13 weeks) and increased risk of congenital anomalies and SABs (Table 1.4) (Miller et al. 1981, Ylinen et al. 1984, Greene et al. 1989, Eidem et al. 2010, Bell et al. 2012).

Table 1.4—Risk of Major Congenital Anomalies in Women with Preexisting Diabetes, by Periconception Glycated Hemoglobin

Periconception Glycated Hemoglobin (%)	Risk of a Pregnancy Affected by Congenital Anomaly (95% CI)	
	Per 1,000 Singleton Pregnancies	For Individual Singleton Pregnancy
5.5	34.3 (8.3, 67.6)	1 in 29 (15, 121)
6.0	30.2 (13.1, 51.0)	1 in 33 (20, 76)
6.1	29.7 (14.3, 48.5)	1 in 34 (21, 70)
6.5	30.3 (18.1, 45.5)	1 in 33 (22, 55)
7.0	38.4 (26.5, 53.1)	1 in 26 (19, 38)
7.5	50.6 (36.8, 66.8)	1 in 20 (15, 27)
8.0	60.1 (45.1, 77.6)	1 in 17 (13, 22)
8.5	72.3 (55.5, 89.3)	1 in 14 (11, 18)
9.0	85.5 (66.7, 105.7)	1 in 12 (9, 15)
9.5	95.3 (74.1, 119.4)	1 in 10 (8, 13)
10.0	107.1 (81.4, 135.4)	1 in 9 (7, 12)
10.5	119.3 (87.2, 152.3)	1 in 8 (7, 11)
11.0	134.9 (95.3, 176.4)	1 in 7 (6, 10)
11.5	144.7 (98.7, 191.4)	1 in 7 (5, 10)
12.0	151.5 (95.2, 206.1)	1 in 7 (5, 11)
12.5	158.9 (90.8, 222.2)	1 in 6 (5, 11)
13.0	167.2 (84.0, 247.4)	1 in 6 (4, 12)
13.5	175.7 (77.8, 271.0)	1 in 6 (4, 13)

Source: Republished with permission of Springer Science and Business Media BV, from Bell R, Gliniania SV, Tennant PWG, Bilous RW, Rankin J. Peri-conception hyperglycaemia and nephropathy are associated with risk of congenital anomaly in women with pre-existing diabetes: a population-based cohort study. *Diabetologia* 2012;55(4):936–947; permission conveyed through Copyright Clearance Center, Inc.

As a result of these findings, high-risk perinatal centers have developed programs for preconceptional management of the woman with diabetes who is planning a pregnancy. Women are evaluated and counseled about the risks of pregnancy, with a particular emphasis on the importance of normalizing blood glucose levels periconceptionally to reduce the risks of delivering an infant with a major birth defect. Studies from these centers have confirmed that normalizing blood glucose levels before and during the early weeks of pregnancy can reduce the risk of SAB or development of major anomalies to near that of the population without diabetes; with preconception care, the estimated reduction in anomalies is 75% (Wahabi et al. 2012). Thus, the prepregnancy counseling and management that emerged in the 1980s have proven to be vital components in the care of the woman with diabetes. The goals of such a program are listed in Table 1.5. A practical method for organizing and implementing a program for preconception care is outlined in this chapter.

Table 1.5—Goals of Prepregnancy Planning Program

- Assessment of a woman's baseline health status
- Obstetric evaluation
- Intensive education of the patient and her family
- Attainment of optimum diabetic control
- Timing and planning of pregnancy

PREPREGNANCY COUNSELING

Prepregnancy counseling for the woman with diabetes ideally should begin at the onset of puberty and continue until menopause, permanent sterilization, or placement of a long-acting reversible contraception device (LARC), thus encompassing all women with diabetes who have childbearing potential. Furthermore, these women should be divided into two categories—those planning a pregnancy within the near future and those wanting to delay pregnancy. For women not currently planning a pregnancy, general information can be given regarding the risks of pregnancy and the importance of appropriate birth control and prepregnancy planning. Physicians should review menstrual history, sexual activity, and contraception plans even among adolescents who have no immediate plans for pregnancy. This is an ideal time to establish a foundation of knowledge and sense of ownership regarding family planning.

For the woman contemplating pregnancy soon, a preconception consultation is essential, and this is the appropriate time to introduce the woman with diabetes to the concept of a healthcare team, assembled to provide the best possible care for diabetic pregnancy. The team consists of physicians, nurses, dietitians, and social workers, all with expertise in this area. The physicians on the team may include an obstetrician or internist with special expertise and interest in diabetic pregnancy, as well as a specialist in maternal-fetal medicine and endocrinology. Other specialists often are included as needed—for example, a nephrologist or ophthalmologist may play a major role when the patient with diabetes has vascular complications. Diabetes nurse educators generally have the greatest amount of contact with the patient, communicating frequently to help with the maintenance of good metabolic control. A neonatologist or pediatrician is poised to provide information to the patient regarding what to expect after the baby is born.

A planned pregnancy is a major objective of preconception counseling; thus, establishing an effective contraceptive method must be an early priority in prepregnancy planning (see Chapter 9). The healthcare provider should review with the woman her options for contraception and help her choose the one most appropriate for her immediate and long-term goals. The healthcare provider should explain to the woman the risks of pregnancy to her developing baby (Table 1.2) as well as to herself (Table 1.1). This prepregnancy counseling session is the ideal moment to emphasize to the woman her two- to fivefold increased risk of having a baby with a congenital anomaly and her increased risk for having a first-trimester SAB if blood glucose levels are not well controlled. Although women can make meaningful improvements in their glucose control after conception, there is insufficient time for this improvement to lead to a significant reduction in congenital anomaly risk. As such, the emphasis must be on normalizing blood glucose levels before pregnancy and continuing this into the early weeks of pregnancy. She should be apprised that organogenesis is largely complete by the 9th week of gestation after her last menstrual period (7th week after conception) and that, with efforts to normalize blood glucose levels before conception, her risk for having a baby with a congenital anomaly or an early SAB can be reduced significantly. Furthermore, she can be assured that with continued optimal glucose control throughout pregnancy, she can effectively reduce her risk of developing further complications.

The healthcare provider should advise the woman of her own personal risks when undertaking pregnancy, emphasizing to her the need for evaluation for the presence of complications resulting from diabetes and other general medical problems before conception. She will need to know that the chronic complications of diabetes can worsen during pregnancy, although debate persists as to whether the pregnancy itself influences the natural course of these complications. Retinopathy has been known to progress in some patients during pregnancy, at approximately double the rate in women who are pregnant compared with women who are not (Morrison et al. 2016). Postpartum regression of retinopathy that worsened during pregnancy is also common but not universal. If the woman has known renal insufficiency or severe gastroenteropathy, she should be advised that these conditions constitute significant risks to both mother and developing infant and, in some individuals, may be relative contraindications to pregnancy. The presence of ischemic heart disease, known to be associated with significant maternal mortality, is in most cases a contraindication to pregnancy.

Genetics is another important aspect of preconception counseling. The woman with diabetes may be reassured that it is rare for a newborn to develop diabetes. If she has T1D and is ≥25 years old, the chance of her child developing T1D at some point is ~1%; if she is <25 years old, this chance increases to ~4% (Warram et al. 1991). If both parents have T1D, the risk is higher, in the range of 10–25% (Warram et al. 1991). T2D is present in ~12% of the adult U.S. population (Centers for Disease Control and Prevention 2017). The risk for offspring of women with T2D to eventually develop T2D ranges from 1 in 7 (14%) when the parent has developed T2D before the age of 50 years old, to 1 in 13 (7.6%) when the onset was later (American Diabetes Association 2018). Although these risks of developing diabetes are higher than that of the general population, they are not significant enough to advise a woman against pregnancy on genetic grounds.

Finally, the healthcare provider must convey to each woman the importance of the deep personal commitment that she will be undertaking during the pregnancy. The demands of maintaining a routine to normalize the blood glucose are many. For some patients, the actual cost of such an undertaking may be prohibitive. The woman needs to understand that once pregnant, she will be seen frequently by her healthcare team, perhaps as often as weekly. She may require hospitalization if problems with the pregnancy develop or her metabolic control deteriorates. She will be undergoing various special tests throughout the pregnancy to assess the well-being of her developing baby. She may want to check with her insurance company to see what coverage her policy offers with regard to pregnancy. Many states offer supplemental aid programs to indigent women during pregnancy. The patient can seek help through her local health department or her state's maternal or child health division.

PREPREGNANCY ASSESSMENT

The prepregnancy assessment (American Diabetes Association 2004, 2019a) of a woman with diabetes (Table 1.6) should begin with a detailed diabetic history, including the following:

- Type of diabetes, including age of onset, duration, and course of disease
- Past history, including hospitalizations for treatment of acute and chronic complications
- Current diabetic regimen, with attention to routine insulin dosages, prior or current use of oral glucose-lowering agents, medical nutrition therapy and individualized meal plan, exercise, hypoglycemia unawareness, and self-monitoring of blood glucose
- History of other medical problems, especially hypertension and thyroid disease
- A careful obstetric history, with attention to contraceptive use and past history of infertility or pregnancy complications, such as hypertensive disease of pregnancy, polyhydramnios, and preterm labor
- All medications that the woman is taking
- A support system, including family and work environment

Table 1.6—Prepregnancy Assessment for Women with Diabetes

- History and physical examination
- Gynecologic evaluation including ensuring cervical cancer screening is up to date
- Laboratory evaluation
  - Prenatal labs, including urinalysis and culture, cervical cultures, blood typing; and screening for rubella, syphilis, hepatitis B virus, and HIV testing
  - Diabetes-specific evaluation, including A1C level, serum creatinine level, thyroid studies, including thyroid-stimulating hormone (TSH) level and spot urinary albumin-to-creatinine ratio
- Smoking cessation as appropriate
- Special studies
- Electrocardiogram if diabetes has been longstanding
- Neuropathy testing if indicated
- Prescription of prenatal vitamin (with at least 400 µg folic acid)
- Initiation of 81 mg aspirin (ASA) at the beginning of second trimester through delivery in women with T1D and T2D to reduce the risk of preeclampsia (American Diabetes Association 2018)

The healthcare provider should perform a careful physical examination with special attention not only to diabetes-related complications, but also to other organ-system abnormalities, especially hypertension. Known hypertension in a woman with diabetes should be treated promptly with medications. In any women considering pregnancy, labetalol, nifedipine, and methyldopa are recommended as first-line agents (ACOG 2013). Angiotensin-converting enzyme (ACE) inhibitors and angiotensin receptor blockers (ARBs) are contraindicated in pregnancy because of their possible teratogenicity and their known association with fetal and neonatal renal failure.

The following are recommendations concerning blood pressure control in pregnancy (ACOG 2013; American Diabetes Association 2019a, 2019b):

- Nonpregnant patients with diabetes who have hypertension should be treated to a blood pressure <140 mmHg systolic and <90 mmHg diastolic; however, lower targets of <130 mmHg systolic and <80 mmHg diastolic may be appropriate in patients with high risk of cardiac disease.
- Pregnant women with diabetes who have chronic hypertension should receive drug therapy when lifestyle and behavioral therapy are not adequate to control blood pressure. Initiation of therapy is not recommended unless systolic blood pressure approaches ≥160 mmHg or diastolic blood pressure approaches ≥105 mmHg (ACOG 2013).
- Drugs safe for pregnancy should be added sequentially until target blood pressure levels are achieved.
- ACE inhibitors and ARBs are contraindicated in pregnancy.
- Women not achieving target blood pressure despite multiple-drug therapy should be referred to a physician experienced in the care of pregnant women with diabetes who have hypertension.
- All women with diabetes, especially those with hypertension, should be monitored closely for the development of preeclampsia.
- 24-h ambulatory blood pressure monitoring or blood pressure self-measurements may provide a more complete picture of the blood pressure burden than isolated office blood pressure measurement and should be considered when determining the need for, or monitoring the effect of, antihypertensive therapy.

Regardless of a woman's blood pressure, all women with T1D and T2D are at risk for chronic renal disease. A serum creatinine and a urinary albumin-to-creatinine ratio should be obtained preconception to screen for undiagnosed renal disease.

All women with T1D or T2D need regular eye exams through dilated pupils by an eye specialist. If this examination reveals pre-proliferative retinopathy or macular edema, proper treatment, including laser photocoagulation, should be performed and the woman's retinal status stabilized before pregnancy. Risk factors for progression of retinopathy include the following:

- Duration of diabetes
- Dyslipidemia
- Kidney disease
- Retinal status
- Elevated A1C
- Rapid normalization of glucose control
- Hypertension
- Valsalva maneuver (increases risk of retinal hemorrhage)

The possible presence of cardiac disease should be evaluated carefully. If a woman has had diabetes for >10 years, or any duration of diabetes and hypertension, the healthcare provider should consider obtaining an electrocardiogram and perhaps even proceed with more in-depth cardiac testing to rule out underlying ischemic heart disease, especially if the woman reveals a history of chest pain.

In addition to this thorough medical assessment, the woman should undergo a careful gynecologic examination. Prompt detection and treatment of gynecologic abnormalities, such as infection or structural deformities, are advantageous. Additionally, it is important to determine from the history whether the woman has any degree of infertility, so that a specific problem can be treated early to minimize any delay for the planned pregnancy.

On completion of the preconception assessment, the patient will see her physician for a return counseling appointment. At that visit, her physician will review with her the results of her tests and discuss her current health status and individualized risk assessment for pregnancy. The discovery of certain diabetes-related complications may serve as relative contraindications for pregnancy (Table 1.7).

Table 1.7 — Potential Contraindications to Pregnancy

- ■ Ischemic heart disease
- ■ Active proliferative retinopathy, untreated
- ■ Renal insufficiency: creatinine clearance <50 mL/min, serum creatinine >1.4 mg/dL, or severe proteinuria (>2 g/24 h)
- ■ Severe gastroenteropathy: nausea or vomiting and diarrhea

If the woman is found to have clinically proven ischemic cardiac disease, the risks of maternal mortality approach 50% with a 30% risk of perinatal loss (Gordon et al. 1996). The woman with this very serious complication should be counseled against undertaking pregnancy, and options for permanent sterilization should be reviewed. If the woman is found to have significant proliferative retinopathy, she should be advised to delay the pregnancy until the ophthalmologist can treat her eye disease appropriately and determine that the retinopathy has stabilized. If she displays significant renal disease (serum creatinine >1.4 mg/dL or creatinine clearance <50 mL/min), she should be counseled about the high risk of morbidity and mortality for her infant that is associated with this particular complication (Biesenbach et al. 1999). Obstetric complications include preeclampsia, premature delivery, small for gestational age/low birth weight, cesarean delivery, and pregnancy loss; of note, odds of preeclampsia and premature delivery were higher in women with nondiabetic nephropathy compared to diabetic nephropathy (Piccoli et al. 2013). Severe gastroenteropathy, in which women are having difficulty maintaining their weight, should be considered a relative contraindication to pregnancy given the risk of severe hypoglycemia and malnutrition if oral intake is not tolerated (Kitzmiller et al. 2008). Metabolic control and nutrition for both the woman and her developing baby are difficult to maintain with this particular complication. In conclusion, if the woman shows no evidence of active diabetic complications or other health problems that place her at significant risk, she may be safely advised to begin plans for pregnancy. At this point, she may be entered into the prepregnancy management protocol.

PREPREGNANCY MANAGEMENT

Once a woman has undergone prepregnancy counseling and assessment, and her individualized risks have been discussed, her healthcare provider should outline a plan for prepregnancy management, the goal of which is to normalize the blood glucose levels before conception and to maintain euglycemia throughout the pregnancy. In achieving preconception goals, the woman with diabetes benefits from effective application of diabetes self-management skills. Members of the management team, which includes diabetes educators and registered dietitians, may provide appropriate education based on assessment, intervention, and monitoring of a woman's response.

Before pregnancy, women with diabetes should be encouraged to adopt a healthy lifestyle, including a healthy diet, moderate to vigorous activity, and emotional well-being. Obesity is an independent risk factor for adverse pregnancy outcomes. Women with diabetes who are overweight (body mass index [BMI] 25–29.9 kg/m^2) or obese (BMI ≥30 kg/m^2) should be encouraged to lose weight. Weight loss can reduce insulin resistance in women who are overweight or obese, assisting glycemic control. Moderate weight loss and cardiovascular disease (CVD) risk reduction may be achieved by balancing caloric intake and physical activity.

The prepregnancy meal plan should meet nutrient recommendations based on the Institute of Medicine's *Dietary Reference Intakes* (DRIs) (Institute of Medicine, Food and Nutrition Board 2006; also see Chapter 3). Caloric needs for women are based on age and physical activity level.

To achieve weight loss, a reduction in caloric intake or an increase in physical activity must occur. Carbohydrate management is a key factor in achieving glucose control and should be individualized. Carbohydrates from fruits, vegetables, whole grains, legumes, and low-fat milk are encouraged to meet nutrient recommendations. A pattern of three meals and some snacks can provide satiety, promote weight goals, and transition to the pregnancy meal plan. Additionally, women with diabetes should do the following:

- Limit saturated fat to <7% of total kcals.
- Minimize intake of trans fats.
- Limit dietary cholesterol to <200 mg/day.
- Reduce sodium intake to 2,300 mg/day.

The 2015–2020 *Dietary Guidelines for Americans* (U.S. Department of Health and Human Services and U.S. Department of Agriculture 2015) recommend that all women in the periconceptional period consume 400 µg/day synthetic folic acid from fortified foods or supplements and additional amounts from a varied diet.

Next, a woman who cannot meet glucose goals through diet should be placed on a multiple injections regimen in a basal-bolus fashion (Table 1.9), or an insulin pump if she is not already practicing an intensive regimen. If the woman has been treated with oral hypoglycemic agents, discontinuation and initiation of insulin therapy should be considered as insulin is the recommended first-line agent for diabetes in pregnancy by all professional societies. Some offer metformin as an alternative, but in preexisting diabetes, it is often inadequate for achieving optimal control.

Insulin is the mainstay of therapy for preexisting diabetes in pregnancy. Intensive insulin therapy with either three or four injections of insulin per day or the use of an insulin pump is necessary in most patients to achieve the near-normal blood glucose goals that are defined in Table 1.8. Both multiple daily injections (MDI) and continuous subcutaneous insulin infusion (CSII) use the concept of basal and bolus insulin replacement to mimic normal physiologic delivery of insulin during fasting and eating. Skills for intensive diabetes self-management are best learned before pregnancy, so that excellent glycemic control is achieved at the time of conception and during organogenesis. Unfortunately, this is not always possible, as approximately 50% of pregnancies are unplanned. A woman's strong motivation to care for her fetus by improving her diabetes control, however, offers a window of opportunity to teach her skills that she may continue to use for the rest of her life.

Table 1.8—Estimated Calories for Women to Achieve Calorie Balance at Different Activity Levels

Age (years)	Sedentary	Moderately Active	Active
19–25	2,000	2,200	2,400
26–45	1,800	2,000	2,200

Source: Adapted from U.S. Department of Health and Human Services and U.S. Department of Agriculture (2015).

If the woman is not familiar with techniques for self-monitoring of blood glucose, these skills should be taught or reviewed (see Chapter 2). She should begin testing her blood glucose levels frequently—before meals and 1 or 2 h after meals—to assess the adequacy of her insulin regimen. Preconception goals for

Table 1.9—Goals for Prepregnancy Daily Insulin Therapy

Goals of therapy

- A1C as close to normal as possible (<7%)
- Fasting capillary plasma glucose <95 mg/dL (5.3 mmol/L)
- 1- or 2-h postprandial capillary plasma glucose <140 mg/dL (<7.8 mmol/L) or <120 mg/dL (<6.7 mmol/L), respectively

Source: Adapted from ACOG (2018), American Diabetes Association (2019a).

fasting capillary glucose levels should be <95 mg/dL (5.3 mmol/L), and 2-h post-meal glucose levels should be <120 mg/dL (<6.7 mmol/L) (ACOG 2018, American Diabetes Association 2019a). On the basis of the record of a woman's self-monitoring of blood glucose, the diabetes team can then prescribe adjustments in diet, insulin, or exercise that will aid her in achieving euglycemia. If the woman is adept and well-motivated, she can learn to make adjustments in her routine at home (American Diabetes Association 2019a).

Eight insulin analogs have been approved by the U.S. Food and Drug Administration (FDA) for use in nonpregnant patients (Table 1.10). Regular insulin, insulin aspart, insulin lispro, NPH (neutral protamine Hagedorn), and detemir have the most data pertaining to use in human pregnancy (Blum 2016). Rapid-acting insulins may improve patient adherence, decrease postmeal glucose excursions, and lower the risk of nocturnal hypoglycemia. Neither lispro nor aspart appears to cross the placenta (Klieger et al. 2008, McCance et al. 2008, Hedrington and Davis 2017). Both lispro and aspart appear to achieve lower 1- to 2-h postprandial glucose levels in women with T1D, T2D, or gestational diabetes mellitus (GDM) compared with regular insulin (Mukerji and Feig 2017).

Basal insulin is used to approximate the fasting insulin requirements. Both long-acting and intermediate-acting insulin can be used as basal insulin immediately before and during pregnancy. With regard to long-acting insulin, two have been studied in pregnancy. Glargine, which does not appear to cross the placenta (Pollex et al. 2010), is associated with a six- to eightfold increase in binding to the IGF receptor and putative mitogenic potency, respectively, compared with regular insulin (Kurtzhals et al. 2000, Ciaraldi et al. 2001). The mitogenic response of insulin relative to IGF-1 is ~1%. Thus, at physiologic concentrations, glargine may not display significant augmentation of mitogenic effects compared with regular insulin. The clinical significance of these binding and mitogenic effects is not known. The long-acting insulin analog glargine (Lantus) provides steady serum levels over 24 h in patients who are not pregnant. Detemir (Levemir), another long-acting insulin, has been recently studied in pregnancy. A randomized controlled trial comparing its use with NPH insulin in pregnancy demonstrated less hypoglycemia with detemir (Mathiesen et al. 2012). Likely as a result, detemir (Levemir) is now an FDA pregnancy category B drug. Despite this recent study, NPH is still frequently used as basal insulin in women planning to conceive in part because NPH can be mixed with short-acting insulin limiting the number of injections a woman must give herself. NPH peaks at 4–8 h and has a duration of action of 10–20 h. Daytime and nighttime hypoglycemia is common in diabetic pregnancies (Kimmerle et al. 1992, Bolli et al. 1993). The relatively short peak action profile of NPH may explain the high risk of nocturnal hypoglycemia, even when taken at bedtime, in the setting of the low fasting glucose treatment goals established for pregnancy. Predinner dosing of intermediate-acting insulin increases the risks of nocturnal hypoglycemia and fasting hyperglycemia but may be reasonable for some patients to simplify the regimen. A bedtime snack usually is needed to reduce this risk. Middle-of-the-night blood glucose levels should be checked occasionally depending on the clinical situation. Ideally, the morning dose of intermediate-acting insulin should be given within 8–10 h after the bedtime dose to avoid hyperglycemia as the nighttime insulin concentration is waning.

An alternative to MDI is CSII. CSII uses a short- or rapid-acting insulin delivered by continuous infusion to deliver a small predetermined amount of insulin per hour. Steady-state basal levels of insulin are achieved. Titration of the basal insulin dose is based on the premeal glucose value. Bolus insulin treatment requires an understanding of medical nutrition therapy. Rapid-acting insulin is given when carbohydrate is ingested. Rapid-acting insulin may be given with a set meal plan that involves consistent carbohydrate at meals and snacks or that is based on a predetermined insulin-to-carbohydrate ratio allowing for more flexible carbohydrate intake. A correction dose based on a calculated sensitivity factor is given to treat an elevated glucose value. Titration of the bolus insulin level is based on the trends of the postprandial glucose value. This approach to bolus insulin is used with both MDI and CSII.

CSII offers multiple programmable basal rates that can be especially useful for patients with nocturnal hypoglycemia and a prominent dawn phenomenon. The disadvantage of CSII is the potential for marked hyperglycemia and diabetic ketoacidosis as a consequence of insulin delivery failure. Although the occurrence is relatively infrequent, this can occur when technical problems arise with the pump, the catheter kinks, an air bubble in the tubing displaces insulin, or accidental displacement occurs at the infusion site. Women who use CSII in pregnancy can take steps to avoid the serious problem of diabetic ketoacidosis by testing blood glucose levels before and after meals, at bedtime, and within 2 h of changing the infusion set. Patients always should test blood glucose levels and ketones if symptoms of hyperglycemia and especially nausea develop, although these symptoms can be masked by pregnancy symptoms. Blood glucose levels >180 mg/dL in the absence of urine ketones should be rechecked within 2 h of a high bolus to ensure that glucose levels are improving. Glucose levels >180 mg/dL in the presence of urine ketones should be treated immediately with a subcutaneous injection. Blood glucose levels and urine ketones should be checked hourly until ketone levels return to normal. The infusion setup should be changed and glucose levels carefully reevaluated.

Inherent in diabetic regimens aimed at normalizing blood glucose levels using insulin is the very real risk of severe hypoglycemia (Kimmerle et al. 1992, Bolli et al. 1993). Before undertaking such a regimen, the woman and her partner should be warned about the risks of hypoglycemia. The diabetes educator should remind them about the signs, symptoms, and management of hypoglycemia, and the partner or a relative should be instructed in the use of glucagon. Proper education about hypoglycemia will result in fewer hospitalizations for this potentially life-threatening complication. The benefits of sensors to warn of hypoglycemia should also be discussed with patients who experience frequent hypoglycemia.

Additionally, instruction in an appropriate exercise routine will enhance the woman's physical fitness and act as an adjunct in maintaining optimal blood glucose control. The woman should also put into practice general principles of good health that may include cessation of smoking, alcohol intake, or unnecessary drugs and medications.

Table 1.10—FDA-Approved Insulins for Use in Pregnancy

Insulin	Time to Onset	Peak Time	Duration	Pregnancy Category
Regular U-100	30 min	3 h	8 h	B
Regular U-500	30 min	3 h	Up to 24 h	B
Aspart	10–15 min	40–50 min	3–5 h	B
Lispro U-100 and U-200	10–15 min	30–90 min	3–5 h	B
Glulisine	10–15 min	55 min	3–5 h	C
NPH	1–2 h	4–8 h	10–20 h	B
Detemir	1–2 h	None	24 h	B
Glargine U-100	1–2 h	None	24 h	No human pregnancy data (previously C)
Glargine U-300	>6 h	None	24 h	No human pregnancy data
Degludec U-100 and U-200	1 h	None	42 h (at steady state)	C
Inhaled human insulin	12–15 min	57 min	2 h	C

Source: Adapted from Blum (2016).

PREVIOUS GESTATIONAL DIABETES MELLITUS

A woman who has had GDM in a previous pregnancy is at significant risk to develop GDM in subsequent pregnancies, as well as T2D in the future. For these reasons, it is important to provide the woman with a past history of GDM with information about these associated risks. Ideally, prepregnancy counseling should begin in the immediate postpartum period, when a woman is still sensitive to the rigors of diabetes management.

The provider can explain to the woman that she has an ~50% chance of developing GDM in future pregnancies (Schwartz et al. 2015), and up to 70% lifetime risk of developing T2D (Kim et al. 2002). Prior pregnancy factors associated with increased risk include early diagnosis of GDM and use of insulin (Rayanagoudar et al. 2016). Current guidelines suggest performing a 2-h, 75-g glucose tolerance test between 4 and 12 weeks postpartum (American Diabetes Association 2019a), but patient compliance and completion of postpartum screening are poor (Eggleston et al. 2016, Werner et al. 2016, Goueslard et al. 2017). Interventions such as phone calls and text message reminders, home visits, and postal mail have demonstrated mixed success (Van Ryswyk et al. 2015, Hamel and Werner 2017). Group prenatal care may improve postpartum visit attendance rates and postpartum diabetes screening (Mazzoni et al. 2016). As a result, screening patients before hospital discharge after delivery has been explored with early promising results, and screening should be further investigated as a reliable alternative (Nabuco et al. 2016, Werner et al. 2016, Carter et al. 2018).

If overt diabetes is discovered early in the postpartum period by the obstetrics team, the patient should be referred to her primary care physician for recommendations on lifestyle changes and possible ongoing medical therapy. Patients who are found to have prediabetes in this period also warrant tremendous efforts by the healthcare team to intervene with lifestyle modifications or metformin to reduce the risk of T2D. Finally, women with normal postpartum screening must be counseled that their risk for diabetes remains elevated compared to women without GDM and that they should complete diabetic screening (fasting plasma glucose, A1C, or 75-g glucose tolerance test) every 1–3 years (American Diabetes Association 2019a).

There is some suggestion that weight reduction before a future pregnancy may reduce the risk of recurrent GDM; thus, if overweight or obese, the woman should be strongly encouraged to lose weight before undertaking another pregnancy (American Diabetes Association 2019a). During this "teachable" period, when she has just experienced the daily commitment required of a person with diabetes, she may be more motivated to follow a weight-reduction plan. If she is willing, she can be referred for dietary counseling.

Finally, the woman should be encouraged to have a yearly follow-up with her healthcare provider. At this session, the provider can determine a fasting glucose level (normal value <100 mg/dL [<5.6 mmol/L]) or A1C (normal value <5.7%), assess success in weight reduction if appropriate, and review pregnancy plans. If there is any suspicion that diabetes has developed in the interim, the patient should be tested appropriately. Subsequent planning for pregnancy will depend on the findings during these annual visits. Of course, if the patient has developed diabetes and desires pregnancy, she should be enrolled immediately in the prepregnancy program described for women with preexisting diabetes (American Diabetes Association 2004, 2019a).

SELECTED READINGS

Alexander EK, Pearce EN, Brent GA, Brown RS, Chen H, Dosiou C, Grobman WA, Laurberg P, Lazarus JH, Mandel SJ, Peeters RP, Sullivan S. Guidelines of the American Thyroid Association for the diagnosis and management of thyroid disease during pregnancy and the postpartum. *Thyroid* 2017;27(3):315–389. PMID: 28056690

Casey BM, Thom EA, Peaceman AM, Varner MW, Sorokin Y, Hirtz DG, Reddy UM, Wapner RJ, Thorp JM, Saade G, Tita ATN, Rouse DJ, et al. for the Eunice Kennedy Shriver National Institute of Child Health and Human Development Maternal–Fetal Medicine Units Network. Treatment of subclinical hypothyroidism or hypothyroxinemia in pregnancy. *N Engl J Med* 2017;376:815–825. PMID: 28249134

Ochsenbein-Kolble N, Roos M, Gasser T, Huch R, Zimmermann R. Cross sectional study of automated blood pressure measurements throughout pregnancy. *Br J Obstet Gynaecol* 2004;111:319–325. PMID: 15008766

Zhang JJ, Ma XX, Hao L, Liu LJ, Lv JC, Zhang H. A systematic review and metaanalysis of outcomes of pregnancy in CKD and CKD outcomes in pregnancy. *Clin J Am Soc Nephrol* 2015;10(11):1964–1978. PMID: 26487769

REFERENCES

American College of Obstetricians and Gynecologists; Task Force on Hypertension in Pregnancy. Hypertension in pregnancy. Report of the American College of Obstetricians and Gynecologists' Task Force on Hypertension in Pregnancy. *Obstet Gynecol* 2013;122(5):1122–1131. PMID: 24150027

American College of Obstetricians and Gynecologists. Practice bulletin no. 190: Gestational diabetes mellitus. *Obstet Gynecol* 2018;131(2):e49–e64. PMID: 29370047

American Diabetes Association. Position statement: preconception care of women with diabetes. *Diabetes Care* 2004;27(Suppl. 1):S76–S78

American Diabetes Association. Genetics of diabetes. Available from www.diabetes.org/diabetes-basics/genetics-of-diabetes.html. Accessed 3 March 2018

American Diabetes Association. Management of diabetes in pregnancy: standards of medical care in diabetes, 2019. *Diabetes Care* 2019a;42(Suppl. 1):S165–S172

American Diabetes Association. Cardiovascular disease and risk management: standards of medical care in diabetes, 2019. *Diabetes Care* 2019b;42(Suppl. 1):S103–S123

Bell R, Glinianaia SV, Tennant PWG, Bilous RW, Rankin J. Peri-conception hyperglycaemia and nephropathy are associated with risk of congenital anomaly in women with pre-existing diabetes: a population-based cohort study. *Diabetologia* 2012;55(4):936–947

Biesenbach G, Grafinger P, Stoger H, Zarzgornik J. How pregnancy influences renal function in nephropathic type 1 diabetic women depends on their preconceptional creatinine clearance. *J Nephrol* 1999;12:41–46. PMID: 10203003

Blum A. Insulin use in pregnancy: an update. *Diabetes Spectr* 2016;29(2):92–97. PMCID: PMC4865394

Bolli GB, Perriello G, Fanelli C, De Feo P. Nocturnal blood glucose control in type 1 diabetes mellitus. *Diabetes Care* 1993;16(Suppl. 3):71–89. PMID: 8299480

Carter EB, Martin S, Temming LA, Colditz GA, Macones GA, Tuuli MG. Early versus 6–12 week postpartum glucose tolerance testing for women with gestational diabetes. *J Perinatol* 2018;38(2):118–121. doi:10.1038/jp.2017.159; PMID: 29048411

Centers for Disease Control and Prevention. National Center for Health Statistics, last updated May 3, 2017. Available from www.cdc.gov/nchs/fastats/diabetes.htm. Accessed 20 February 2019

Ciaraldi TP, Carter L, Seipke G, Mudaliar S, Henry RR. Effects of the long-acting insulin glargine on cultured human skeletal muscle cells: comparisons to insulin and IGF-1. *J Clin Endocrinol Metab* 2001;86:5838–5847. PMID: 11739448

Diabetes Control and Complications Trial Research Group. Pregnancy outcomes in the Diabetes Control and Complications Trial. *Am J Obstet Gynecol* 1996;174(4):1343–1353. PMID: 8623868

Eggleston EM, LeCates RF, Zhang F, Wharam JF, Ross-Degnan D, Oken E. Variation in postpartum glycemic screening in women with a history of gestational diabetes mellitus. *Obstet Gynecol* 2016;128(1):159–167. PMID: 27275787

Eidem I, Stene LC, Henriksen T, Hanssen KF, Vangen S, Vollset SE, Joner G. Congenital anomalies in newborns of women with type 1 diabetes: nationwide population-based study in Norway, 1999–2004. *Acta Obstet Gynecol Scand* 2010;89:1403–1411. PMID: 20929418

Evers IM, de Valk HW, Visser GH. Risk of complications of pregnancy in women with type 1 diabetes: nationwide prospective study in the Netherlands. *BMJ* 2004;328(7445):915. PMID: 15066886

Freinkel N, Lewis NJ, Akazawa S, Roth S, Forman L. The honeybee syndrome: implications of the teratogenicity of mannose in rat-embryo culture. *N Engl J Med* 1984;310:223–230. PMID: 6690398

Gordon MC, Landon MB, Boyle J, Stewart KS, Gabbe SG. Coronary artery disease in insulin-dependent diabetes mellitus of pregnancy (class H): a review of the literature. *Obstet Gynecol Surv* 1996;51(7):437–444. PMID: 8807644

Greene MF. Prevention and diagnosis of congenital anomalies in diabetic pregnancy. *Clin Perinatol* 1993;20:533–547. PMID: 8222466

Greene MF, Hare JW, Cloherty JP, Benacerraf BR, Soeldner JS. First-trimester hemoglobin A1C and risk for major malformation and spontaneous abortion in diabetic pregnancy. *Teratology* 1989;39:225–231. PMID: 2727930

Goueslard K, Cottenet J, Mariet A, Sagot P, Petit JM, Quantin C. Early screening for type 2 diabetes following gestational diabetes mellitus in France: hardly any impact of the 2010 guidelines. *Acta Diabetol* 2017;54(7):645–651. PMID: 28393277

Hamel MS, Werner EF. Interventions to improve rate of diabetes testing postpartum in women with gestational diabetes mellitus. *Curr Diab Rep* 2017;17(2):7. PMID: 28150160

Hare JW, White P. Pregnancy in diabetes complicated by vascular disease. *Diabetes* 1977;26:953–955. PMID: 908464

Hedrington MS, Davis SN. The care of pregestational and gestational diabetes and drug metabolism considerations. *Expert Opin Drug Metab Toxicol* 2017;13(10):1029–1038. PMID: 28847172

Institute of Medicine, Food and Nutrition Board. *Dietary Reference Intakes: The Essential Guide to Nutrient Requirements*. Washington, DC, National Academies Press, 2006

Kalter H, Warkany J. Congenital malformations: etiologic factors and their role in prevention. *N Engl J Med* 1983;308:424–431. PMID: 6337330

Kim C, Newton KM, Knopp RH. Gestational diabetes and the incidence of type 2 diabetes: a systematic review. *Diabetes Care* 2002;25(10):1862–1868. PMID: 12351492

Kimmerle R, Heinemann L, Delecki A, Berger M. Severe hypoglycemia: incidence and predisposing factors in 85 pregnancies of type 1 diabetic women. *Diabetes Care* 1992;15:1034–1037. PMID: 1505305

Kitzmiller JL, Block JM, Brown FM, Catalano PM, Conway DL, Coustan DR, Gunderson EP, Herman WH, Hoffman LD, Inturrisi M, Jovanovic LB, Kjos SI, Knopp RH, Montoro MN, Ogata ES, Paramsothy P, Reader DM, Rosenn BM, Thomas AM, Kirkman MS. Managing preexisting diabetes for pregnancy: summary of evidence and consensus recommendations for care. *Diabetes Care* 2008;31(5):1060–1079. PMID: 18445730

Kitzmiller JL, Cloherty JP, Younger MD, Tabatabaii A, Rothchild S, Sosenko I, Epstein M, Sinah S, Neff R. Diabetic pregnancy and perinatal outcome. *Am J Obstet Gynecol* 1978;131:560–580. PMID: 354386

Klieger C, Pollex E, Koren G. Treating the mother–protecting the unborn: the safety of hypoglycemic drugs in pregnancy. *J Matern Fetal Neonatal Med* 2008;21(3):191–196. PMID: 18297574

Kurtzhals P, Schaffer L, Sorensen A, Kristensen C, Jonassen I, Schmid C, Trüb T. Correlations of receptor binding and metabolic and mitogenic potencies of insulin analogs designed for clinical use. *Diabetes* 2000;49:999–1005. PMID: 10866053

Macintosh MC, Fleming KM, Bailey JA, Doyle P, Modder J, Acolet D, Golightly S, Miller A. Perinatal mortality and congenital anomalies in babies of women with type 1 or type 2 diabetes in England, Wales, and Northern Ireland: population based study. *BMJ* 2006;333(7560):177. PMID: 16782722

Mathiesen ER, Hod M, Ivanisevic M, et al., on behalf of the Detemir in Pregnancy Study Group. Maternal efficacy and safety outcomes in a randomized, controlled trial comparing insulin detemir with NPH insulin in 310 pregnant women with type 1 diabetes. *Diabetes Care* 2012;35(10):2012–2017. PMID: 22851598

Mazzoni SE, Hill PK, Webster KW, Heinrichs GA, Hoffman MC. Group prenatal care for women with gestational diabetes. *J Matern Fetal Neonatal Med* 2016;29(17):2852–2856. PMID: 26461437

McCance DR, Damm P, Mathiesen ER, Hod M, Kaaja R, Dunne F, Jensen LE, Mersebach H. Evaluation of insulin antibodies and placental transfer of insulin aspart in pregnant women with type 1 diabetes mellitus. *Diabetologia* 2008;51:2141–2143. PMID: 18726086

Miller E, Hare JW, Cloherty JP, Dunn PH, Gleason RE, Soeldner JS, Kitzmiller JL. Elevated maternal hemoglobin A1c in early pregnancy and major congenital anomalies in infants of diabetic mothers. *N Engl J Med* 1981;304:1331–1134. PMID: 7012627

Mills JL, Baker L, Goldman AS. Malformations in infants of diabetic mothers occur before the seventh gestational week: implications for treatment. *Diabetes* 1979;28:292–293. PMID: 437367

Miodovnik M, Lavin JP, Knowles HC, Holroyde J, Stys S. Spontaneous abortion among insulin-dependent diabetic women. *Am J Obstet Gynecol* 1984;150:372–375. PMID: 6207729

Morrison JL, Hodgson LA, Lim LL, Al-Qureshi S. Diabetic retinopathy in pregnancy: a review. *Clin Exp Opthalmol* 2016;44(4):321–334. PMID: 27062093

Mukerji G, Feig DS. Pharmacological management of gestational diabetes mellitus. *Drugs* 2017;77:1723–1732. PMID: 28864965

Nabuco A, Pimentel S, Cabizuca CA, Rodacki M, Finamore D, Oliveira MM, Zajdenverg L. Early diabetes screening in women with previous gestational diabetes: a new insight. *Diabetol Metab Syndr* 2016;8(1):61. PMID: 27570545

Piccoli GB, Clari R, Ghiotto S, Castelluccia N, Colombi N, Mauro G, Tavassoli E, Melluzza C, Cabiddu G, Gernone G, Mongilardi E, Ferraresi M, Rolfo A, Todros T. Type 1 diabetes, diabetic nephropathy, and pregnancy: a systematic review and meta-study. *Rev Diabet Stud* 2013;10(1):6–26. PMID: 24172695

Pollex EK, Feig DS, Lubetsky A, Yip PM, Koren G. Insulin glargine safety in pregnancy: a transplacental transfer study. *Diabetes Care* 2010;33:29–33. PMID: 19808914

Rayanagoudar G, Hashi AA, Zamora J, Khan KS, Hitman GA, Thangaratinam S. Quantification of the type 2 diabetes risk in women with gestational diabetes: a systematic review and meta-analysis of 95,750 women. *Diabetologia* 2016;59(7):1403–1411. PMID: 27073002

Reece EA, Gabriella S, Abdalla M. The prevention of diabetes associated birth defects. *Semin Perinatol* 1988;12:292–302. PMID: 3065942

Reece EA, Hobbins JS. Diabetic embryopathy: pathogenesis, prenatal diagnosis and prevention. *Obstet Gynecol Surv* 1986;41:325–335. PMID: 2423939

Sadler TW, Hunter ES, Wynn RE, Phillips LH. Evidence for multifactorial origin of diabetes-induced embryopathies. *Diabetes* 1989;38:70–74. PMID: 2909414

Schwartz N, Nachum Z, Green MS. The prevalence of gestational diabetes mellitus recurrence—effect of ethnicity and parity: a metaanalysis. *Am J Obstet Gynecol* 2015;213(3):310–317. PMID: 25757637

U.S. Department of Health and Human Services and U.S. Department of Agriculture. *2015–2020 Dietary Guidelines for Americans.* 8th ed. December 2015. Available from http://health.gov/dietaryguidelines/2015/guidelines/. Accessed 8 March 2018

Van Ryswyk EM, Middleton PF, Hague WM, Crowther CA. Postpartum SMS reminders to women who have experienced gestational diabetes to test for type 2 diabetes: the DIAMIND randomized trial. *Diabet Med* 2015;32(10): 1368–1376. PMID: 25816702

Wahabi HA, Alzeidan RA, Esmaeil SA. Pre-pregnancy care for women with pre-gestational diabetes mellitus: a systematic review and meta-analysis. *BMC Public Health* 2012;12:792. PMID: 2297874

Warram JH, Martin BC, Krowlewski AS. Risk of IDDM in children of diabetic mothers decreases with increasing maternal age at pregnancy. *Diabetes* 1991;40:1679–1684. PMID: 1756908

Watkins ML, Rasmussen SA, Honein MA, Botto LD, Moore CA. Maternal obesity and risk for birth defects. *Pediatrics* 2003;111(5Pt2):1152–1158. PMID: 12728129

Werner EF, Has P, Tarabulsi G, Lee J, Satin A. Early postpartum glucose testing in women with gestational diabetes mellitus. *Am J Perinatol* 2016;33(10): 966–971. PMID: 27120481

Ylinen K, Aula P, Stenman U-H, Kesaniemi-Kuokkanea T, Teramo K. Risk of minor and major fetal malformations in diabetics with high haemoglobin A1c values in early pregnancy. *BMJ* 1984;289:345–346. PMID: 6432090

Zabihi S, Loeken MR. Understanding diabetic teratogenesis: where are we now and where are we going? *Birth Defects Res A Clin Mol Teratol* 2010;88(10): 779–790. PMCID: PMC5070114

Assessment of Glycemic Control

Highlights
Assessment of Glycemic Control

■ Hyperglycemia is the major cause of complications of diabetes and pregnancy. Normoglycemia minimizes these complications.

■ Self-monitoring of blood glucose (SMBG) is a key component of diabetes therapy during pregnancy in women with type 1 diabetes, type 2 diabetes, and gestational diabetes mellitus and should be included in the management plan. Daily SMBG with capillary blood glucose sampling at least 3–4 times a day will provide optimal results in pregnancy.

■ Finger-stick SMBG testing is preferable in pregnancy, as alternative site testing may not identify rapid changes in blood glucose concentrations characteristic of pregnant women with preexisting diabetes.

■ Routinely evaluate the patient's technique and ability to use SMBG data to adjust therapy.

■ The American Congress of Obstetricians and Gynecologists and American Diabetes Association recommend treatment targets of preprandial glucose <95 mg/dL and postprandial <140 mg/dL at 1 h or 120 mg/dL at 2 h, although lower mean glucose values may further reduce the risk of pregnancy complications.

■ The use of continuous interstitial glucose monitoring, while promising, needs more evaluation before it can be recommended for general use in pregnant women with diabetes.

Assessment of Glycemic Control

Pregnancy is a complex endocrine and metabolic state involving impaired insulin sensitivity; compensatory pancreatic β-cell insulin secretion; moderately increased blood glucose levels; and changes in levels of circulating free fatty acids, triglycerides, cholesterol, and phospholipids. This physiologic change ensures that fetal, placental, and maternal energy demands are met (Di Cianni et al. 2003). To understand the pathologic state of diabetes in pregnancy, we must first elucidate the patterns of normoglycemia in healthy pregnancies.

Studies of intermittent capillary blood glucose and continuous interstitial glucose monitoring in normal pregnant women have revealed a consistent and predictable range of glucose concentrations. In a study summarizing data from eleven investigations spanning three decades, patterns of glycemia in the third trimester (mean gestational age 33.8 ±2.3 weeks; range 24–40.8 ±0.09–8.1 weeks) were graphed (Figure 2.1) (Hernandez et al. 2011). The study incorporated subjects in both inpatient and outpatient settings who were monitored using either intermittent SMBG or continuous interstitial glucose monitoring. On average, blood glucose was 70.9 ±8 mg/dL at fasting, and 96–122 and 89–110 mg/dL at 1- and 2-h postprandial, respectively.

The effect of gestational age on patterns of normoglycemia has also been evaluated. Fasting plasma glucose concentrations decline modestly, by ~2 mg/dL, in early normal pregnancy (Mills et al. 1998), with a slight, gradual rise in mean and postprandial glucose values throughout the second and third trimesters of normal pregnancy.

These studies elucidating normoglycemic states in pregnancy have called into question the current goals set by the American College of Obstetricians and Gynecologists (ACOG) and American Diabetes Association in patients with diabetes in pregnancy, which recommend treatment targets of fasting <95 mg/dL and postprandial <140 mg/dL at 1 h or 120 mg/dL at 2 h (American Diabetes Association 2017, ACOG 2018). Recent data from the Hyperglycemia and Adverse Pregnancy Outcomes (HAPO) study suggest that concentrations of maternal glucose, even below these currently accepted cut-offs, have a strong, continuous association with increased birth weight and increased cord-blood serum C-peptide levels (Metzger et al. 2008). To date, there are no adequately powered randomized controlled trials (RCTs) comparing different glycemic targets in diabetes in pregnancy.

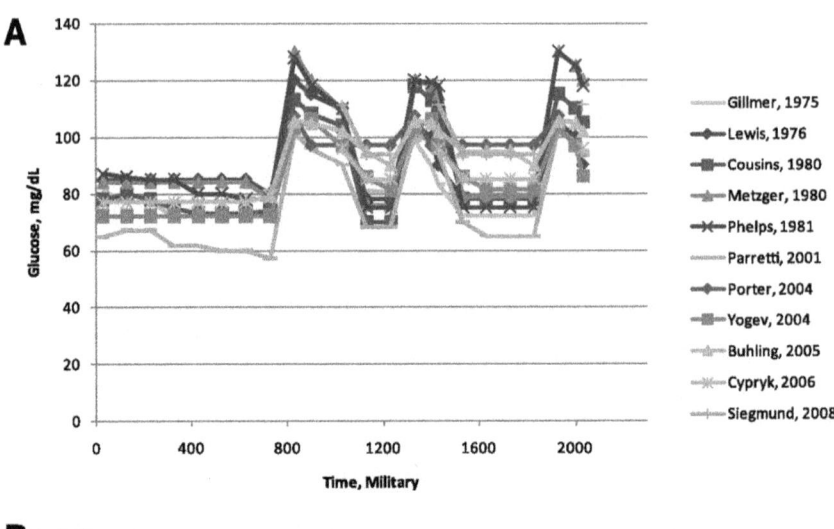

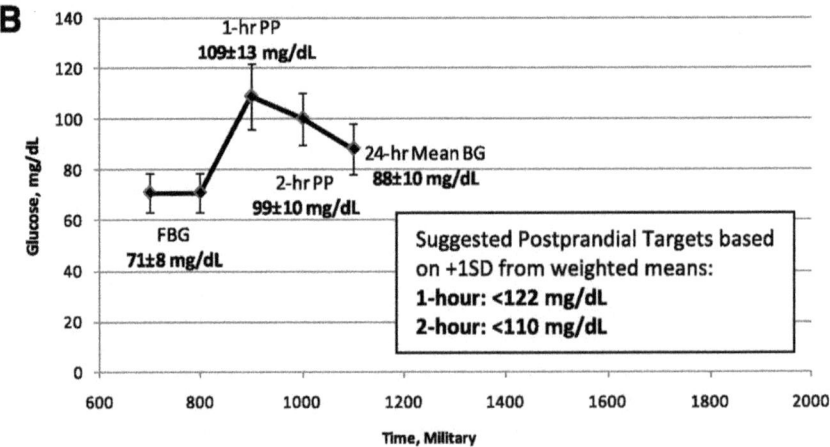

Figure 2.1—A: Patterns of glycemia in normal third-trimester pregnancies across 11 studies published between 1975 and 2008 and **B:** suggested postprandial targets.

Source: Hernandez et al. (2011).

SELF-MONITORING OF CAPILLARY BLOOD GLUCOSE

Self-monitoring of blood glucose (SMBG) is an integral part of the intensified treatment of diabetes that has dramatically improved pregnancy outcome over the past 25 years (Sacks et al. 2002, American Diabetes Association 2018). Self-monitoring allows pregnant women and their healthcare providers to determine the most effective therapeutic modality and dosage (e.g., diet, physical activity, or insulin) to control glucose levels (Negrato and Zajdenverg 2012). Adherence to SMBG protocols as recommended by the American Diabetes Association and ACOG is associated with clinically and statistically better glycemic control regardless of diabetes type or therapy (Karter et al. 2001).

SITE OF SMBG

To provide less discomfort with glucose self-testing, manufacturers developed products designed for use at alternative sites—usually the forearm or thigh (American Diabetes Association 2011). When glucose concentrations are rapidly rising or falling (e.g., postprandially, immediately after exercise, or with insulin-induced hypoglycemia), however, there is a lag time of 15–30 min between the finger-stick capillary glucose concentration and the alternative site testing of the forearm and thigh (Ellison et al. 2002, Jungheim and Koschinsky 2002, Bina et al. 2003). This lag time is further exaggerated with low temperatures because of decreased perfusion (Haupt et al. 2005). Therefore, use of alternative site testing systems in the dynamic state of pregnancy will give different results than finger-stick testing (American Diabetes Association 2018) and is not recommended. Palm and fingertip capillary glucose values are similar at different time points (Bina et al. 2003, Meguro et al. 2005), but these testing sites have not been compared in pregnancy.

TIMING OF SMBG

Conventional intensified glucose monitoring is defined by the American Diabetes Association as three to four blood glucose measurements per day (American Diabetes Association 2018). Postprandial glucose levels have been shown to be a better predictor of fetal macrosomia than preprandial levels in observational studies (Jovanovic et al. 1991, Combs et al. 1992, Parretti et al. 2003, Moy et al. 2014). An RCT of preprandial versus postprandial glucose testing in gestational diabetes mellitus (GDM) reported lower frequencies of perinatal complications with treatment strategies based on postmeal results (de Veciana et al. 1995). A similar result was found in an RCT of preprandial versus postprandial testing starting at 16 weeks of gestation in women with type 1 diabetes (T1D) (Manderson et al. 2003).

Although SMBG recommendations in patients who are not pregnant utilize preprandial glucose values, SMBG protocols in pregnancy focus on blood glucose after meals (American Diabetes Association 2018). Postprandial blood glucose can be assessed at either 1 or 2 h after initiation of meals (ACOG 2018). The choice of timing should reflect the peak and nadir of maternal glucose levels. Studies with continuous interstitial glucose monitoring in pregnant women with diabetes show the mean peak postprandial glucose to average 90 min after beginning the meal, with considerable variation from patient to patient (Ben-Haroush et al. 2004) and high day-to-day variability (Kerssen et al. 2004a). Factors that affect timing and extent of postprandial glucose excursions include delayed gastric emptying (Stanley et al. 1995), timing of the meals (Sivan et al. 2001), and fat or protein content and glycemic index of meals (Bell et al. 2015, Paterson et al. 2015).

The pharmacokinetic profile of the treatment should also be considered. Initially, 2-h postprandial testing was utilized because of the actions of regular insulin, with effect peaking at approximately 2–3 h after injection. Rapid-acting insulin analogs have peak effect at ~60 min after injection, so testing at 1-h postprandial may better guide medication titration (American Diabetes Association 2015).

Both the American Diabetes Association and ACOG recommend that the fasting or preprandial glucose value be <95 mg/dL and the postprandial glucose value be <140 mg/dL at 1 h and 120 mg/dL at 2 h to reduce the risk of macrosomia. These values are reviewed on a weekly basis by the provider, with adjustments to frequency of testing based on number of excursions (ACOG 2018). As mentioned previously, no controlled trials have been conducted to evaluate optimal glycemic targets in pregnancy.

Note that preprandial values also may continue to play a role in management of patients with pregestational diabetes, who use the information to determine the dosage of short-acting or rapid-acting insulin injections before meals (American Diabetes Association 2018). Bedtime and overnight blood levels also can be assessed as needed to guide recommendations on lifestyle changes or insulin doses.

CONTINUOUS GLUCOSE MONITORING IN PREGNANCY

Continuous glucose monitoring (CGM) devices measure subcutaneous interstitial tissue glucose by an electrochemical method, usually at 5- to 10-s intervals with values reported as averages over 5 min, yielding an average of 288 values per day. (Hewapathirana et al. 2013). CGM technology has been extensively studied in patients who are not pregnant over the past two decades and has been shown to improve hemoglobin A_{1c} (A1C) levels in adults who are not pregnant and children without increased hypoglycemia (Polsky and Garcetti 2017).

Two types of CGM exist: real-time CGM (rtCGM) provides near real-time glucose data and alarms for excursions, whereas intermittent CGM (iCGM) shows measurements retrospectively at the time of data review. Although the American Diabetes Association recommends CGM use in pregnancy for some high-risk women, such as those with hypoglycemia unawareness (Kitzmiller et al. 2008), its broader clinical utility in all pregnant patients with preexisting diabetes continues to be debated. Feasibility studies of CGM systems in pregnancies of women with T1D revealed periods of both hyper- and hypoglycemia that were not detected by traditional SMBG or patient symptoms (Yogev et al. 2003a, 2003b; Ben-Haroush et al. 2004; Kerssen et al. 2004b, 2006). Among RCTs of continuous glucose monitoring in pregnancies complicated by T1D and type 2 diabetes (T2D), some studies have found CGM to be associated with improved glycemic control in the third trimester, lower birth weight, reduced risk of macrosomia, and improved neonatal outcomes (Murphy et al. 2008, Feig et al. 2017), whereas other RCTs have found no difference in maternal and neonatal outcomes (Secher et al. 2013, Polsky and Garcetti 2017). More prospective studies or meta-analyses are needed to ascertain whether application of this technology to pregnancies complicated by T1D and T2D will improve perinatal outcome and maternal safety.

Providers must remind patients that interstitial glucose readings also can be affected by acetaminophen use, particularly in those sensors measuring hydrogen peroxide (Zhang et al. 1994). Additional barriers to successful CGM use include discomfort, sensor accuracy, pharmacologic interference with readings, cost, reimbursement issues, and lack of time and training for healthcare professionals (Polsky and Garcetti 2017).

FACTORS AFFECTING GLUCOSE LEVELS

Whether using capillary glucose monitoring or interstitial glucose monitoring, it is important to remember that numerous factors affect maternal glucose levels, including the following:

- Stress (physical stress in the form of trauma, inflammation, infection, or hormonal imbalance due to growth and development, menstrual cycle, or pregnancy; exogenously administered steroids; and psychological stress)
- Time of day
- Exercise
- Amount of carbohydrate eaten

Stress, both psychological and physical, increases blood glucose levels via the sympathoadrenal hormones cortisol and adrenaline, similar to outside of pregnancy. Pregnancy-related hormonal effects from cortisol, progesterone, and human placental lactogen, however, exacerbate the normal phenomenon of morning glucose intolerance. For this reason, hyperglycemia after breakfast commonly occurs in GDM unless carbohydrate intake is restricted. Typically, greater percentages of carbohydrate can be tolerated later in the day. The time of day also affects blood glucose levels because of the diurnal variation of contra-insulin hormones. Middle-of-the-night hypoglycemia in the first trimester in particular is common for women with T1D. Consistency in the meal plan with an evening snack can reduce this risk.

Exercise can also significantly affect glucose levels in women regardless of type of diabetes. Even low-impact exercise decreases blood glucose levels by increasing the uptake of glucose into the cells without extra insulin. Although exercise tends to increase the risk of hypoglycemia, carbohydrates affect the risk of hyperglycemia. Seminal studies demonstrated that the amount of carbohydrate consumed in a meal or snack is highly correlated with the effect on blood glucose (Peterson 1991, Major 1998). Not all carbohydrates are alike in terms of glycemic properties, however. Choosing higher-quality carbohydrates with a reduced ability to acutely raise blood glucose, such as legumes, whole grains, and vegetables, can optimize micronutrient intake while still controlling glycemia to within treatment targets (Hernandez et al. 2018; see also Chapter 3).

OTHER MEASURES OF METABOLIC CONTROL

Glycated hemoglobin is the general term used to describe a series of stable minor hemoglobin components formed slowly and nonenzymatically in direct proportion to the ambient glucose concentration (Sacks et al. 2002, American Diabetes Association 2018). Glycated hemoglobin values expressed as the percentage of total hemoglobin provide the best assessment of the degree of chronic glycemic control, reflecting the average blood glucose concentration during the preceding 6–12 weeks. In pregnancy, however, it is important to remember that glycated hemoglobin may reflect a shorter time window because the red blood cell life is shortened to <90 days in pregnancy (Lurie and Danon 1992). The value of glycated hemoglobin is also limited in patients with frequent low and high blood glucose levels, as their mean glucose value may approach normal and therefore their glycated hemoglobin will be deceivingly normal and would not reflect postprandial elevations or preprandial deficits (Derr et al. 2003, Kerssen et al. 2007).

Many glycated hemoglobin assays are available, but A1C has become the preferred standard for assessing glycemic control (Sacks et al. 2002, American Diabetes Association 2018). Conditions that may affect A1C levels include hemoglobin variants or states of increased red blood cell turnover (Table 2.1). A list of specific assay interferences by hemoglobinopathies can be found via the NGSP website (2010). Therefore, an A1C result that is different than expected by patient report of SMBG, higher than 15%, or radically different from a previous A1C result from a different lab should trigger a query of the patient's history or laboratory technique utilized (American Diabetes Association 2018).

Table 2.1—Factors That Can Affect A1C Results

Hemoglobinopathies*
- Hemoglobin S
- Hemoglobin E
- Hemoglobin C
- Hemoglobin D
- Elevated levels of hemoglobin F

Increased red blood cell turnover
- Sickle cell disease
- Pregnancy
- Hemodialysis
- Blood loss
- Transfusion
- Erythropoietin therapy

* A list of specific assay interferences by hemoglobinopathies can be found on the NGSP website (NGSP 2010).

Knowledge of A1C levels can aid in management of patients throughout the continuum of pregnancy. Preconception care for women with T1D or T2D is effective in improving rates of congenital malformations, improving perinatal mortality, and reducing maternal A1C in the first trimester of pregnancy (Wahabi et al. 2012). In women with suboptimally controlled maternal blood glucose, rapid correction of hyperglycemia can lead to significant decrease of A1C within 2 weeks of initiation of therapy. Thus, the measurement of A1C every 2–4 weeks can be considered in a selected group of high-risk patients to confirm reported SMBG measurements and provide positive feedback (Jovanovic et al. 2011). The HAPO study, however, suggests that for diagnosis of diabetes, the A1C measurement is not a satisfactory alternative to a screening oral glucose tolerance test in women without preexisting diabetes (Lowe et al. 2012).

Although glycated serum protein assays, such as fructosamine, can be used in patients with hemoglobinopathies, fructosamine has not proved to be useful in pregnancies complicated by diabetes (Sacks et al. 2002, American Diabetes Association 2018). No standardized, published correlation exists between fructosamine levels and mean blood glucose as there is with A1C. Fructosamine theoretically reflects average blood glucose over the past week because of the rapid turnover rate of albumin (8 days in pregnancy). Inaccurate results can arise because of the presence of reducing agents in the patient's blood, such as with vitamin C from prenatal vitamins (Danese et al. 2015). In addition, there is a diurnal variation in serum protein concentrations in the blood. Thus, the woman must have her fructosamine test at the same time of day for each determination or the variation in total serum proteins may be greater than the change in this measure of average blood glucose concentrations.

KETONURIA AND KETONEMIA

Pregnancy is a ketogenic state. Under fasting conditions, fatty acids are converted into ketone bodies throughout the β-oxidation pathway, and these compounds easily cross the placental barrier and are metabolized by the fetus (Herrera 2000). Women with T1D, and to a lesser extent T2D, are at risk for diabetic ketoacidosis at lower blood glucose levels than in the nonpregnant state (Whiteman et al. 1996, Montoro 2004, American Diabetes Association 2018). Testing of urine ketones should be done periodically when a pregnant woman with diabetes is ill, vomiting, or has blood glucose values >200 mg/dL (Whiteman et al. 1996, Kitzmiller et al. 2008).

Table 2.2—Findings in Diabetic Ketoacidosis

Signs and Symptoms	Laboratory Findings
■ Hyperventilation–tachypnea ■ Sinus tachycardia ■ Hypotension or dehydration ■ Change in sensorium, disorientation, or coma ■ Kussmaul respirations or fruity breath ■ Nonreassuring fetal tracing ■ Polyuria or polydipsia ■ Nausea or vomiting ■ Abdominal pain or contractions ■ Blurred vision ■ Muscle weakness	■ Plasma glucose level (nonpregnant: >250 mg/dL; pregnant: >180–200 mg/dL)* ■ Arterial pH less than 7.30* ■ Anion gap greater than 12 mEq/L* ■ Elevated base deficit* ■ Positive serum/urine ketones, especially 3β-hydroxybutyrate (most abundant) ■ Falsely normal serum potassium level might be present ■ Low serum bicarbonate (often less than 15 mEq/L) ■ Elevated serum blood urea nitrogen and creatinine resulting from dehydration and possible renal failure

* These values are variable.

Source: Republished with permission of Wolters Kluwer Health, from Sibai B, Viteri O. Diabetic ketoacidosis in pregnancy. *Obstet Gynecol* 2014;123(1):167–178; permission conveyed through Copyright Clearance Center, Inc.

Diabetic ketoacidosis (DKA) is associated with a high mortality rate in the fetus (Montoro 2004). In addition, fasting ketonemia in pregnant diabetic and nondiabetic women has been associated with decreased intelligence and fine motor skills in offspring (Rizzo et al. 1991). Signs and symptoms and laboratory findings for DKA are listed in Table 2.2.

Patients can keep ketone strips at home and receive education on detection and prevention of diabetic ketoacidosis. Women with moderate to large ketonuria associated with hyperglycemia should alert their physician immediately for a determination of ketonemia and serum electrolytes. Urine ketone tests are not reliable for the firm diagnosis of DKA, which is better made with blood ketone testing that quantifies β-hydroxybutyric acid (Sacks et al. 2002, American Diabetes Association 2018). Home tests for β-hydroxybutyric acid are available, but they have not been evaluated systematically in pregnancy (Kitzmiller et al. 2008).

SELECTED READING

American College of Obstetricians and Gynecologists. Practice bulletin no. 60: Pregestational diabetes mellitus. *Obstet Gynecol* 2005;105:675–685 (reaffirmed 2010)

REFERENCES

American College of Obstetricians and Gynecologists. Practice bulletin no. 180: Gestational diabetes mellitus. *Obstet Gynecol* 2018;131:e49–e64

American Diabetes Association. Position statement executive summary: tests of glycemia in diabetes. *Diabetes Care* 2011;34(Suppl. 1):S1419–S1423

American Diabetes Association. Management of diabetes in pregnancy. *Diabetes Care* 2017;40(Suppl. 1):S114–S119

American Diabetes Association. Insulin basics. Available from http://www.diabetes.org/living-with-diabetes/treatment-and-care/medication/insulin/insulin-basics.html. Last edited 2015. Accessed March 2018

American Diabetes Association. Classification and diagnosis of diabetes: standards of medical care in diabetes, 2018. *Diabetes Care* 2018;41(Suppl. 1):S13–S27

Bell KJ, Smart CE, Steil GM, Brand-Miller JC, King B, Wolpert HA. Impact of fat, protein, and glycemic index on postprandial glucose control in type 1 diabetes: implications for intensive diabetes management in the continuous glucose monitoring era. *Diabetes Care* 2015;38(6):1008–1015

Ben-Haroush A, Yogev Y, Chen R, Rosenn B, Hod M, Langer O. The postprandial glucose profile in the diabetic pregnancy. *Am J Obstet Gynecol* 2004;191:576–581

Bina DM, Anderson RL, Johnson ML, Bergenstal RM, Kendall DM. Clinical impact of prandial state, exercise, and site preparation on the equivalence of alternative-site blood glucose testing. *Diabetes Care* 2003;26:981–985

Combs CA, Gunderson E, Kitzmiller JL, Gavin LA, Main EK. Relationship of fetal macrosomia to maternal postprandial glucose control during pregnancy. *Diabetes Care* 1992;15:1251–1257

Danese E, Montagnana M, Nouvenne A, Lippi G. Advantages and pitfalls of fructosamine and glycated albumin in the diagnosis and treatment of diabetes. *J Diabetes Sci Technol* 2015;9(2):169–176

Derr R, Garrett E, Stacy GA, Suadek CD. Is HbA1c affected by glycemic instability? *Diabetes Care* 2003;26:2728–2733

Di Cianni G, Micooli R, Volpe L, et al. Intermediate metabolism in normal pregnancy and in pregnancy complicated by gestational diabetes. *Diab Metab Res Rev* 2003;19:259–270

de Veciana M, Major CA, Morgan MA, Asrat T, Toohey JS, Lien JM, Evans AT. Postprandial versus preprandial blood glucose monitoring in women with gestational diabetes mellitus requiring insulin therapy. *N Engl J Med* 1995;333: 1237–1241

Ellison JM, Stegman JM, Colner SL, Michael RH, Sharma MK, Ervin KR, Horwitz DL. Rapid changes in postprandial blood glucose produce concentration differences at finger, forearm, and thigh sampling sites. *Diabetes Care* 2002;25:961–964

Feig DS, Donovan LE, Corcoy R, et al. Continuous glucose monitoring in pregnant women with type 1 diabetes (CONCEPTT): a multicenter international randomised controlled trial. *Lancet* 2017;390(10110):2347–2359

Haupt A, Berg B, Paschen P, Dreyer M, Haring HU, Smedegaard J, Matthaei S. The effects of skin temperature and testing site on blood glucose measurements taken by a modern blood glucose monitoring device. *Diabetes Technol Ther* 2005;7(4):597–601

Hernandez TL, Friedman JE, Van Pelt RE, Barbour LA. Patterns of glycemia in normal pregnancy: should the current therapeutic targets be challenged? *Diabetes Care* 2011;34:1660–1668

Hernandez TL, Mande A, Barbour LA. Nutrition therapy within and beyond gestational diabetes. *Diab Res Clin Pract* 2018;145:39–50

Herrera E. Metabolic adaptations in pregnancy and their implications for the availability of substrate to the fetus. *Eur J Clin Nutr* 2000;54(Suppl. 1):S47–S51

Hewapathirana NM, O'Sullivan E, Murphy HR. Role of continuous glucose monitoring in the management of diabetic pregnancy. *Curr Diabetes Rep* 2013;13(1):34–42

Jovanovic L, Peterson CM, Reed GF, Metzger BE, Mills JL, Knopp RH, Aarons JH. Maternal postprandial glucose levels and infant birth weight: the Diabetes in Early Pregnancy Study. The National Institute of Child Health and Human Development—Diabetes in Early Pregnancy Study. *Am J Obstet Gynecol* 1991;164:103–111

Jovanovic L, Savas H, Mehta M, Trujillo A, Pettitt DJ. Frequent monitoring of A1C during pregnancy as a treatment tool to guide therapy. *Diabetes Care* 2011;34(1):53–54

Jungheim K, Koschinsky T. Glucose monitoring in the arm: risky delays of hypoglycemia and hyperglycemia detection. *Diabetes Care* 2002;25:956–960

Karter AJ, Ackerson LM, Darbinian JA, D'Agostino RB, Ferrara A, Liu J, Selby JV. Self-monitoring of blood glucose levels and glycemic control: the Northern California Kaiser Permanente Diabetes registry. *Am J Med* 2001;111(1):1–9

Kerssen A, de Valk HW, Visser GH. Day-to-day glucose variability during pregnancy in women with type 1 diabetes mellitus: glucose profiles measured with the continuous glucose monitoring system. *BJOG* 2004a;111:919–924

Kerssen A, de Valk HW, Visser GH. The continuous glucose monitoring system during pregnancy of women with type 1 diabetes mellitus: accuracy assessment. *Diabetes Technol Ther* 2004b;6:645–651

Kerssen A, de Valk HW, Visser GH. Do HbA1c levels and the self-monitoring of blood glucose levels adequately reflect glycemic control during pregnancy in women with type 1 diabetes mellitus? *Diabetologia* 2006;49:25–28

Kerssen A, de Valk HW, Visser GH. Increased second trimester maternal glucose levels are related to extreme large-for-gestational age infants in women with type 1 diabetes mellitus. *Diabetes Care* 2007;30:1069–1074

Kitzmiller JL, Block JM, Brown FM, et al. Managing preexisting diabetes for pregnancy: summary of evidence and consensus recommendations for care. *Diabetes Care* 2008;31:1060–1079

Lowe LP, Metzger BE, Dyer AR, et al., for the HAPO Study Cooperative Research Group. Hyperglycemia and Adverse Pregnancy Outcome (HAPO) study: associations of maternal A1C and glucose with pregnancy outcomes. *Diabetes Care* 2012;35:574–580

Lurie S, Danon D. Life span of erythrocytes in late pregnancy. *Obstet Gynecol* 1992;80:123–126

Manderson JG, Patterson CC, Hadden DR, Traub AI, Ennis C, McCance DR. Preprandial versus postprandial blood glucose monitoring in type 1 diabetic pregnancy: a randomized controlled clinical trial. *Am J Obstet Gynecol* 2003;189:507–512

Meguro S, Funae O, Hosokawa K, Atsumi Y. Hypoglycemia detection rate differs among blood glucose monitoring sites. *Diabetes Care* 2005;28:708–709

Metzger BE, Lowe LP, Dyer AR, et al., HAPO Study Cooperative Research Group. Hyperglycemia and adverse pregnancy outcomes. *N Engl J Med* 2008;358:1991–2002

Mills JL, Jovanovic, L, Knopp R, Aarons J, Conley M, Park E, Lee YJ, Holmes L, Simpson JL, Metzger B. Physiological reduction in fasting blood glucose concentration in the first trimester of normal pregnancy: the Diabetes in Early Pregnancy Study. *Metabolism* 1998;47:1140–1144

Montoro MN. Diabetic ketoacidosis in pregnancy. In *Diabetes in Women: Adolescence, Pregnancy, and Menopause.* 3rd ed. Reece EA, Coustan DR, Gabbe SG, Eds. Philadelphia, PA, Lippincott Williams & Wilkins, 2004, p. 345–350

Moy FM, Ray A, Buckley BS. Techniques of monitoring blood glucose during pregnancy for women with pre-existing diabetes. *Cochrane Database Syst Rev* 2014;30(4):CD009613

Murphy HR, Rayman G, Lewis K, Kelly S, Johal B, Duffield K, Fowler D, Campbell PJ, Temple RC. Effectiveness of continuous glucose monitoring in pregnant women with diabetes: randomised clinical trial. *BMJ* 2008; 337:a1680

Negrato CA, Zajdenverg L. Self-monitoring of blood glucose during pregnancy: indications and limitations. *Diabetology Metab Synd* 2012;4:54

NGSP. HbA1c Assay Interferences. Copyright 2010. Available from http://www.ngsp.org/interf.asp. Accessed 13 May 2019

Parretti E, Carignani L, Cioni R, Bartoli E, Borri P, La Torre P, Mecacci F, Martini E, Scarselli G, Mello G. Sonographic evaluation of fetal growth and body composition in women with different degrees of normal glucose metabolism. *Diabetes Care* 2003;26:2741–2748

Paterson M, Bell KJ, O'Connell SM, Smart CE, Shafat A, King B. The role of dietary protein and fat in glycaemic control in type 1 diabetes: implications for intensive diabetes management *Curr Diabetes Rep* 2015;15:61

Polsky S, Garcetti R. CGM, pregnancy and remote monitoring. *Diabetes Technol Ther* 2017;19(Suppl. 3):S49–S59

Rizzo T, Metzger BE, Burns WJ, Burns K. Correlations between antepartum maternal metabolism and child intelligence. *N Engl J Med* 1991;325:911–916

Sacks DB, Arnold M, Bakris GL, et al. Guidelines and recommendations for laboratory analysis in the diagnosis and management of diabetes mellitus (Position Statement). *Diabetes Care* 2002;25:750–786

Secher AL, Ringholm L, Andersen HU, et al. The effect of real-time continuous glucose monitoring in pregnant women with diabetes: a randomized controlled trial. *Diabetes Care* 2013;36:1877–1883

Sibai B, Viteri O. Diabetic ketoacidosis in pregnancy. *Obstet Gynecol* 2014;123(1): 167–178

Sivan E, Weisz B, Homko CJ, Reece EA, Schiff E. One or two hours postprandial glucose measurements: are they the same? *Am J Obstet Gynecol* 2001;185: 604–607

Stanley K, Magides A, Arnot M, Bruce C, Reilly C, McFee A, Fraser R. Delayed gastric emptying as a factor in delayed postprandial glycemic response in pregnancy. *Brit J Obstet Gynecol* 1995;102:288–291

Wahabi HA, Alzeidan RA, Esmaeli SA. Pre-pregnancy care for women with pregestational diabetes mellitus: a systematic review and meta-analysis. *BMC Public Health* 2012;12:792

Whiteman VE, Homko CJ, Reece EA. Management of hypoglycemia and diabetic ketoacidosis in pregnancy. *Obstet Gynecol Clinics N Am* 1996;23:87–107

Yogev Y, Ben-Haroush A, Chen R, Kaplan B, Phillip M, Hod M. Continuous glucose monitoring for treatment adjustment in diabetic pregnancies: a pilot study. *Diabet Med* 2003a;20:558–562

Yogev Y, Chen R, Ben-Haroush A, Phillip M, Jovanovic L, Hod M. Continuous glucose monitoring for the evaluation of gravid women with type 1 diabetes mellitus. *Obstet Gynecol* 2003b;101:633–638

Zhang Y, Hu Y, Wilson GS, Moatti-Sirat D, Poitout V, Reach G. Elimination of the acetaminophen interference in an implantable glucose sensor. *Anal Chem* 1994;66:1183–1188

Lifestyle Management for Diabetes in Pregnancy

Highlights
Lifestyle Management for Diabetes in Pregnancy

■ Weight gain recommendations are individualized, based on the Institute of Medicine's revised body mass index (BMI) categories.

■ Most successful models of care include a multidisciplinary team with the woman with diabetes at the center.

■ Medical nutrition therapy should be provided by a registered dietitian or a qualified nutritionist and should include an individualized meal plan.

■ Nutrient needs of pregnant women with diabetes are based on the Institute of Medicine's 2006 *Dietary Reference Intakes*, summarized in Table 3.2.

Lifestyle Management for Diabetes in Pregnancy

WEIGHT GAIN RECOMMENDATIONS

Gaining the appropriate amount of weight during pregnancy enhances maternal and fetal well-being, while avoiding excessive postpartum weight retention, which can have implications for the long-term health of women and their children. Women who become pregnant today do so at a higher body weight than in the past. In fact, in the U.S., less than half of young women (20–39 years old) are normal-weight, and 37% of women of childbearing age are obese (BMI ≥30 kg/m²) (Flegal et al. 2016, Deputy et al. 2018). Studies continue to demonstrate that a woman's pregravid weight and gestational weight gain affect perinatal outcomes (Kitzmiller et al. 2008, Dennedy et al. 2012, Nicklas and Barbour 2015, Barbour and Hernandez 2018). The Institute of Medicine (IOM) recommendations (Table 3.1) evaluate weight gain during pregnancy from the perspective that factors affecting pregnancy begin before conception and continue through the first year after delivery. The weight gain guidelines are based on revised BMI categories and now have a specific recommendation for obese women. To meet the recommendations of the guidelines, women need to gain within the weight gain ranges for their BMI category.

Table 3.1—Institute of Medicine Recommendations for Rate of Weight Gain in Pregnancy

Prepregnancy BMI (kg/m²)	Total Weight Gain (lb)	Rates of Weight Gain Second and Third Trimesters (lb/week)
Underweight (<18.5)	28–40	1 (1–1.3)
Normal weight (18.5–24.9)	25–35	1 (0.8–1)
Overweight (25.0–29.9)	15–25	0.6 (0.5–0.7)
Obese (≥30.0)	11–20	0.5 (0.4–0.6)

Source: Adapted from Institute of Medicine, National Research Council (2009).

Timing and rate of weight gain also affect outcomes. In the first trimester, relatively small amounts of weight gain are required (1.1–4.4 lb) (IOM 2009). In women who do not have diabetes, weight gain in the first half of pregnancy is a determinant of fetal linear growth. In the second and third trimesters, inadequate weight gain in normal-weight and underweight women without diabetes may be associated with premature birth or small-for-gestational-age (SGA) babies. In overweight and obese women, excessive weight gain is associated with an increased rate of fetal macrosomia, birth trauma, and cesarean sections (Kitzmiller et al. 2008, Nicklas and Barbour 2015, Buschur et al. 2018). In women with diabetes, excessive weight gain can promote fetal overgrowth and fat deposition, and has been associated with an increase in cesarean deliveries. It has been suggested that women with diabetes target weight gain totals at the lower end of the IOM's recommended weight gain range for BMI category. Weight loss is not recommended, but women with diabetes who are obese and consuming adequate calories and nutrients (as evidenced by review of detailed food records) may not need to reach minimum weight gain recommendations (IOM 1990). More research is needed in pregnant women with diabetes to determine the effects of pregravid BMI, gestational weight gain, and weight retention on perinatal outcomes.

Many BMI calculators are available online (Centers for Disease Control and Prevention 2018). Height and weight should be measured at the first prenatal visit (American College of Obstetricians and Gynecologists [ACOG] 2015b). Care should be taken to assess height accurately, but pregravid weight status is often subjective information. An accurate height–weight history may be available from health records and can be supportive data. If the woman with diabetes has had preconception counseling, this information may be more readily available. When reported pregravid weight is not reasonable based on current weight and gestational age, an estimated weight can be utilized. BMI category can then be assigned. Weight should be monitored at each visit (ACOG 2015b, American Diabetes Association 2018). Patterns of gain can be plotted using prenatal weight gain grids based on the IOM's recommended ranges. This tool can be used to educate and motivate the pregnant woman with diabetes to engage in efforts to gain the appropriate amounts of weight (see Selected Readings). Women who have gained excessive amounts of weight early in gestation should not be severely restricted, but weight gain may be slowed and weight loss should be encouraged for the postpartum period (Kitzmiller et al. 2008).

CONTROVERSY: CALORIE RESTRICTION FOR OBESE PATIENTS

In 2009, the IOM revised its recommendations for weight gain during pregnancy (IOM 2009). Women of normal prepregnancy weight (BMI 18.5–24.9 kg/m^2) are advised to gain 25–35 lb; those who are overweight (BMI 25–29.9 kg/m^2) are advised to gain 15–25 lb; and obese individuals (BMI >30 kg/m^2) are advised to gain 11–20 lb. This was the first time that the IOM included upper limits for weight gain in pregnancy. A recent area of interest is the use of hypocaloric diets for obese women with gestational diabetes mellitus (GDM). One study indicated that restricting calories by 30–33% resulted in reduced hyperglycemia, reduced plasma triglycerides, and no increase in ketonuria, whereas a 50% reduction in caloric intake was associated with ketonuria (Knopp et al. 1991). Other studies showed that calorie restriction (1,200–1,800 calories/day) normalized birth weights in babies of mothers with GDM with no increase in perinatal morbidity, although urinary ketones were not measured (Dornhorst et al. 1991). Also, fewer women required insulin. One explanation for these results is that the women experienced an improvement in insulin sensitivity secondary to calorie restriction. The women in this study gained only 1.7 ±1.6 kg (3.7 ±3.5 lb) during the third trimester. Another potential advantage of calorie restriction is reduced postpartum obesity. The calorie-restricted approach might decrease the concentration of all maternal fuels reaching the fetal circulation (amino acids, plasma triglyceride fatty acids, and glucose), thereby reducing macrosomia. Levels of free fatty acids and ketones may increase, however, so further research is needed to determine whether calorie restriction might adversely affect the future health of the infant. In an observational study of 223 pregnant women (preexisting diabetes 40%; GDM 44%; normal glucose metabolism 16%), third-trimester β-hydroxybutyrate levels, which did not differ among the three groups, correlated inversely with mental development index scores in the offspring at 2 years of age and with Stanford-Binet scores at 3–5 years of age (Rizzo et al. 1991). Moreover, a recent prospective trial linked gestational weight gain ≤5 kg in overweight or obese women with an increased risk of SGA (Catalano et al. 2014), a finding also corroborated by a meta-analysis of 13 studies across 437,512 obese women (Xu et al. 2017). Such data give pause to efforts to impose caloric restriction in pregnancy severe enough to cause elevated ketone levels.

Currently, no method has been scientifically validated to estimate energy requirements in overweight and obese women. In clinical practice and some research protocols, the caloric prescription used for obese women is 25 kcal/kg and for normal-weight women is 35 kcal/kg based on prepregnancy weight (Diabetes Care and Education Practice Group 2007). Some practitioners use the Harris Benedict equation (with adjustments), and some use in-depth nutrition assessment, weight history, and clinical judgment. No matter the method used, the monitoring of nutrient adequacy, weight-gain patterns, and blood glucose levels should be ongoing and adjusted based on outcome measures.

NUTRITIONAL MANAGEMENT IN PREGNANCY

FOR PREEXISTING DIABETES

Nutrition is one of the most important influences on the health of pregnant women and their infants. Maintaining a good nutritional status optimizes maternal health, reduces the risk of birth defects and suboptimal fetal growth, and lowers the risk of chronic health problems in their children (American Dietetic Association [now Academy of Nutrition and Dietetics] 2008). In pregnant women with preexisting diabetes, excellent glucose control from the first trimester and continued throughout pregnancy is associated with the lowest frequency of maternal, fetal, and neonatal complications (Kitzmiller et al. 2008). Optimal glucose control, both before and early in pregnancy, has been shown to improve perinatal outcomes (Jovanovic et al. 2005). Historically, population surveys looking at infants of women with type 1 diabetes (T1D) indicated an excessive rate of macrosomia (birth weight >4,000 g or >4,500 g) compared with the general population (Johnstone et al. 2006), an observation that continues in the contemporary environment on a background of increasing incidence of T1D (Wahabi et al. 2012).

The profound effects of changes in maternal metabolism during pregnancy on women with diabetes necessitate intensive management. The most successful models of care include a multidisciplinary team with the woman with diabetes at the center (Kitzmiller et al. 2008). Individualized medical nutrition therapy (MNT) should be provided, preferably by a registered dietitian or qualified nutritionist with knowledge of MNT specific to pregnancy and diabetes (Every 2013, Kitzmiller et al. 2008, American Diabetes Association 2018). All members of the clinical team should understand and support the individualized meal plan. The pregnant woman should be a primary active member of the treatment team. The diabetes management team may guide, educate, and support the pregnant woman with diabetes, but she must manage her diet, perform self-monitoring of blood glucose (SMBG) levels, and keep extensive records. Pregnant women often are excited and motivated to make healthy lifestyle changes for their developing baby. Pregnancy visits can provide an opportunity to educate the woman with diabetes to adjust her diet to reduce the risk of, or to better manage, concurrent complications of preexisting diabetes and improve long-term health.

The goals of MNT for pregnancy in women with preexisting diabetes are to provide adequate nutrients for maternal and fetal needs while minimizing pregnancy complications, to promote appropriate weight gain, and to maintain optimal glucose control (Kitzmiller et al. 2008, Evert et al. 2014, Buschur et al. 2018). The current nutrient requirements for pregnant women with diabetes are similar to those for the pregnant population without diabetes and are based on the Dietary Reference Intakes (DRIs), which are summarized in the IOM's *Dietary Reference Intakes: The Essential Guide to Nutrient Requirements* (IOM 2006). DRIs for nonpregnant, pregnant, and lactating women are given in Table 3.2.

Table 3.2—Dietary Reference Intakes for Women[a]

Nutrient	Adult Woman	Pregnancy	Lactation (0–6 months)
Energy (kcal)	2,403	2,743[b], 2,855[c]	2,698
Protein (g/kg/d)	0.8	1.1	1.1
Carbohydrate (g/d)	130	175	210
Total fiber (g/d)	25	28	29
Fluids, l/day (cups/d)	2.2 (~9)	2.3 (~10)	3.1 (~13)
Linoleic acid (g/d)	12	13	13
α-Linolenic acid (g/d)	12	13	13
Vitamin A (μg RAE)	700	770	1,300
Vitamin D (μg)[d,e]	10	10	10
Vitamin E (mg α-tocopherol)	15	15	19

Table 3.2 (continued)

Nutrient	Adult Woman	Pregnancy	Lactation (0–6 months)
Vitamin K (µg)	90	90	90
Vitamin C (mg)	75	85	120
Thiamin (mg)	1.1	1.4	1.4
Riboflavin (mg)	1.1	1.4	1.6
Vitamin B_6 (mg)	1.3	1.9	2.0
Niacin (mg NE)[f]	14	18	17
Folate (µg dietary folate equivalents)	400	600	500
Vitamin B_{12} (µg)	2.4	2.6	2.8
Pantothenic acid (mg)	5	6	7
Biotin (µg)	30	30	35
Choline (mg)	425	450	550
Calcium (mg)	1,000	1,000	1,000
Phosphorus (mg)	700	700	700
Magnesium (mg)	320	350	310
Iron (mg)	18	27	19
Zinc (mg)	8	11	12
Iodine (µg)	150	220	290
Selenium (µg)	55	60	70
Fluoride (mg)	3	3	3
Manganese (mg)	1.8	2.0	2.6
Molybdenum (µg)	45	50	50
Chromium (µg)	25	30	45
Copper (µg)	900	1,000	1,300
Sodium (mg)	2,300	2,300	2,300
Potassium (mg)	4,700	4,700	5,100

RAE, retinol activity equivalents.

[a] Values are recommended dietary average requirements except energy (estimated energy requirement) and total fiber, linoleic acid, α-linolenic acid, vitamin K, pantothenic acid, biotin, choline, manganese, chromium, sodium, and potassium, in which cases the recommended adequate intake is noted.

[b] Second trimester for women ages 19–50 years old.

[c] Third trimester for women ages 19–50 years old.

[d] As cholecalciferol: 1 µg cholecalciferol = 40 IU vitamin D.

[e] Under the assumption of minimal sunlight.

[f] NE = niacin equivalents: 1 mg niacin = 60 mg tryptophan.

Source: Data from Institute of Medicine, Food and Nutrition Board (2006, 2010).

FOR GESTATIONAL DIABETES MELLITUS

MNT is the cornerstone to management of all women with GDM and is based on the standard nutritional recommendations for pregnant women. The principles are similar to those for pregnant women with preexisting diabetes. All women with GDM should receive nutritional counseling by a registered dietitian or qualified nutritionist when possible. In the management of GDM, MNT provided by a registered dietitian or nutritionist results in decreased hospital admissions and insulin use, improves the likelihood of normal fetal and placental growth, and reduces the risk of perinatal complications, especially when diagnosed and treated early. Initial interventions should occur as soon as possible after diagnosis (within 1 week) and should include follow-up visits (Reader et al. 2006, Academy of Nutrition and Dietetics 2017). Individualization of MNT depending on maternal weight and height is recommended (Evert et al. 2014, American Diabetes Association 2018). The goals of MNT in GDM are as follows:

- Achieve and maintain normoglycemia, most typically defined as fasting plasma glucose ≤95 mg/dL (≤5.3 mmol/L), 1-h postprandial plasma glucose ≤140 mg/dL (≤7.8 mmol/L), and 2-h postprandial plasma glucose ≤120 mg/dL (≤6.7 mmol/L).
- Provide a nutritionally adequate diet for pregnancy. A nutritionally adequate, balanced diet contains all the essential nutrients required for fetal development and maintenance of maternal health. It also provides sufficient calories for the woman to achieve an appropriate weight gain and for her to avoid ketonuria.

INDIVIDUALIZED MEAL PLANNING AND RECORDKEEPING

Meal plans for women with diabetes in pregnancy must be developed on an individual basis, based on the nutritional assessment of the patient. This plan should promote a balanced diet that takes into account ethnic, cultural, and financial concerns (American Diabetes Association 2018, Hernandez et al. 2018). A qualified educator, preferably a registered dietitian, should teach the patient, emphasizing appropriate portion sizes. Next, the educator should determine the appropriate calorie level and the amount of carbohydrate, protein, and fat for the individual using the basics shown in Table 3.3. The educator then should record the number of servings from each food group to include in the daily diet. With the patient, the educator needs to develop a sample menu. To verify that the patient understands the meal plan, the patient should be asked to plan another sample menu, using a resource such as *Choose Your Foods: Food Lists for Diabetes*.

Many programs recommend three meals and three snacks, regardless of whether or not the patient is taking insulin. Others feel that an overweight patient achieves better glucose control by simply consuming three meals and a bedtime snack (to prevent nocturnal ketone production). Snacks can be advantageous because protein-containing snacks between meals prevent extreme hunger at the next meal, and smaller meals and snacks every few hours are easier for pregnant women to digest.

Table 3.3—Basic Meal Plan for Pregnancy and Lactation

Food Group	Minimum No. Daily Servings
Whole-grain breads, rice, pasta, cereal	6–9 servings
Vegetables (include green leafy and yellow)	4 servings
Fruits (include vitamin C source daily)	3 servings
Milk, cheese, yogurt (low fat)	3 servings
Meat, fish, poultry (lean), dry beans, eggs, and nuts	2 servings
Oils (includes fat from nuts)	6 tsp

Source: Adapted from U.S. Department of Agriculture, Center for Nutrition Policy and Promotion (2010).

Overall, meal plans for pregnant women with diabetes focus on consistency and advocating small dietary changes (Table 3.4). Macronutrients, including carbohydrate, are distributed throughout the day.

Keeping daily food logs in combination with blood glucose logs can provide invaluable information to tailor meal plans and optimize treatment. Checking blood glucose four times a day is recommended and a food log can be charted at those times:

- Fasting (after rising)
- 1 or 2 h after breakfast
- 1 or 2 h after lunch
- 1 or 2 h after dinner

The diet prescription should be validated with SMBG. The diet only "fits" if postprandial hyperglycemia results are low (1-h postprandial blood glucose <140 mg/dL or 2-h values <120 mg/dL). The food records also help the registered dietitian to know whether the patient understands the diet. The records should be evaluated at every visit to provide vital feedback to the patient. These records are important for the following reasons:

- Individual food sensitivities can be pinpointed (e.g., foods that yield a high glycemic response).
- They allow the registered dietitian or nutritionist to evaluate the patient's understanding of the meal plan and to provide appropriate continuing education.
- Perhaps most important, they help the patient learn to make decisions about meal planning.

For women with type 2 diabetes (T2D) and GDM, avoiding hyperglycemia is the primary goal of dietary changes; however, for women with T1D, goals of dietary management include avoiding hypoglycemia. Because of fetal demands for glucose, the pregnant woman may become hypoglycemic if she delays meals, skips a snack or meal, eats too little, exercises more than usual, or takes too much insulin. Hypoglycemia in the first trimester in particular is common for women with T1D. Consistency in the meal plan can minimize this risk.

Table 3.4—Basic Dietary Guidelines: Dos and Don'ts

Guideline	Rationale
Avoid concentrated sweets.	These foods cause hyperglycemia and are usually high in calories and low in nutrients. Emphasize fresh foods.
Avoid highly processed foods.	Eating highly processed foods usually results in a more rapid rise in blood glucose than fresh or less processed foods. Highly processed foods are often high in fat, contributing to excessive weight gain.
Eat small meals.	Consuming small frequent meals helps women avoid postprandial hyperglycemia and preprandial starvation ketosis. A consistent meal pattern is important: three meals and three snacks usually are recommended. Snacks prevent women from becoming overly hungry and overeating at the next meal. Protein foods are encouraged because they are digested and absorbed more slowly than carbohydrates, yielding a lower glycemic response. The fat in protein foods contributes to a greater satiety value than carbohydrate-rich foods, preventing excessive hunger. The small frequent meal pattern also helps to alleviate nausea and heartburn, two common discomforts of pregnancy.
Avoid fruits and juices at breakfast.	Fruits and juices often cause hyperglycemia and should be avoided; milk should be limited (or omitted if postprandial hyperglycemia results).
Eat free foods as desired (celery, lettuce, broccoli, cauliflower, nopales cactus, asparagus, tomatoes).	These foods provide <20 kcal/serving, are very low in carbohydrate, and may be eaten when patients are hungry. These foods can be prepared as soups or eaten raw as salads.

MACRONUTRIENTS

Adequate intake of energy from carbohydrate, fiber, protein, and fat is necessary to support fetal-placental growth and provide for maternal needs and fat storage. These nutrients also have a strong impact on glucose control and pregnancy success for women with diabetes.

The IOM's DRIs are the recommended guidelines for nutrient intake for all stages of the life cycle, including pregnancy (IOM 2006). Values are provided for individual macro- and micronutrients in Table 3.2. Note that women eat foods, not nutrients in isolation. Incorporating a woman's food preferences and tolerances, while encouraging consumption of a wholesome balanced meal plan, is a key component of MNT for pregnant women with diabetes.

ENERGY

Most pregnant women need between 2,200 kcal and 2,900 kcal a day to meet their nutritional needs (American Dietetic Association [now Academy of Nutrition and Dietetics] 2008). This amount should be adjusted taking into consideration prepregnancy BMI, rate of weight gain, maternal age, and appetite (Tables 3.5 and 3.6). Energy requirements for pregnancy are based on the estimated energy requirements of women who are not pregnant with adjustments for pregnancy (IOM 2006).

Table 3.5—Estimated Energy Requirement (kcal/day) Formula

Physical Activity	Physical Activity Coefficient	Activity Examples
Sedentary	1.0	Daily living activities (e.g., household tasks, walking to the bus)
Low active	1.12	Daily living activities + 30–60 min daily moderate activity (e.g., walking at 5–7 km/h)
Active	1.27	Daily living activities + at least 60 min daily moderate activity
Very active	1.45	Daily living activities + 60 min daily moderate activity + additional 60 min of strenuous activity, or 120 min of moderate activity

Estimated energy requirements = [354 – (6.91 × age [years]) + PA* × [(9.36 × weight [kg]) + (726 × height [m])] for nonpregnant women 19–50 years old.
Source: Adapted from Institute of Medicine, Food and Nutrition Board (2006).

Table 3.6—Estimated Energy Requirements Adjusted for Pregnancy

Trimester	Energy Requirements
First trimester	EER + 0 kcal/day
Second trimester	EER + 340 kcal/day
Third trimester	EER + 452 kcal/day

EER, estimated energy requirements.
Source: Adapted from Institute of Medicine, Food and Nutrition Board (2006).

Energy needs may be highly variable and an individualized approach is recommended (Kitzmiller et al. 2008, Evert et al. 2014, American Diabetes Association 2018). With the prevalence of obesity and the importance of controlled weight gain, some women with diabetes in pregnancy may benefit from a reduced energy intake. Studies based on women with GDM have reported good outcomes with energy intakes of 1,700–1,800 kcal/day (limitation of 30%) (Dornhurst et al. 1991). Moderately limiting energy also may be beneficial for women with T2D who are obese and with insulin resistance. More severe restrictions of

1,200–1,600 kcal may lead to weight loss or starvation ketosis, which is of high concern and should be avoided (Knopp et al. 1991, Buschur et al. 2018, Hernandez et al. 2018). Close monitoring of interval weight gains can allow for the adjustment of the energy level of the meal plan. If weight gains are below or above the target range, a discussion should be initiated with the patient regarding an action plan to adjust energy intake and physical activity.

CARBOHYDRATE

Glucose is the preferred fuel for fetal growth and development. Carbohydrate is the primary nutrient affecting maternal glucose levels. The recommended daily allowance (RDA) for an adult woman is 130 g/day of digestible carbohydrate based on the minimum amounts of glucose utilized by the brain. Minimum carbohydrate recommendations for pregnant women increase to 175 g/day to meet fetal needs, particularly brain development (IOM 2005, 2006), but these recommendations do not account for placental glucose requirements, which new evidence suggests likely exceed 135 g alone in the third trimester (Holme et al. 2015, Hernandez et al. 2018). Carbohydrates (i.e., sugars, starches, and fiber) are found in fruits, vegetables, whole grains, legumes, milk, and yogurt, and in the added sugars in the foods we consume. The IOM, Food and Nutrition Board has set the acceptable macronutrient distribution range for carbohydrate for all populations, including pregnant women, at 45–65% of total calories. In women with diabetes, carbohydrate frequently is limited to 40–60% of total calories to meet postprandial blood glucose goals, but it should include the minimum recommendation of 175 g/day of digestible carbohydrate (Kitzmiller et al. 2008). It may be difficult to meet the other nutritional needs of pregnancy when carbohydrate is limited to the minimum requirement. The amount of carbohydrate should be individualized based on patient preferences; weight gain goals; insulin doses; and premeal, postmeal, and nighttime glucose values (American Diabetes Association 2018).

The type of carbohydrate consumed also affects postprandial blood glucose levels. Extrinsic variables may influence postprandial blood glucose values, including fasting or preprandial blood glucose levels, macronutrient distribution of foods consumed, available insulin, and insulin resistance. To meet the nutrient needs of pregnancy, meals and snacks usually include a combination of macronutrients, not only carbohydrate. Use of sucrose in a diabetes meal plan is acceptable (Evert et al. 2014); in pregnancy, however, this should be limited because of the importance of a nutrient-dense diet and weight management. Use of sugar alcohols is permissible, but because sugar alcohols are harder for the body to digest, their effect on blood glucose levels is less than standard sugar. When counting carbohydrates for products made with sugar alcohols, half of the grams of carbohydrates from sugar alcohol should be used to calculate the total carbohydrate load (Knopp et al. 1991).

Women with diabetes can use a variety of methods to manage their carbohydrate intake. Some women "count" carbohydrate grams, some use portion sizes or "exchanges," some estimate portions based on experience or "my plate," and some use a combination of methods. A carbohydrate "choice/exchange" typically has 15 g of carbohydrate. Daytime snacks usually are needed to prevent premeal low blood glucose levels, and an adequate bedtime snack may reduce nocturnal hypoglycemia. Women on intensive management, after education, may use carbohydrate-to-insulin ratios to help manage blood glucose levels. The ratios need frequent adjustment as glucose tolerance varies with gestational age. According to the *Managing Preexisting Diabetes and Pregnancy* (Kitzmiller et al. 2008), carbohydrate distribution for a typical meal plan for a pregnant woman with diabetes would include the following:

- Breakfast: 15–45 g carbohydrate
- Lunch: 30–75 g carbohydrate
- Dinner: 30–75 g carbohydrate
- Daytime snacks: 15–30 g carbohydrate
- Bedtime snack: 15–45 g carbohydrate

Close monitoring of food and SMBG records by the management team can help a woman meet her goals of excellent glycemia, adequate nutrients, and appropriate weight gain.

DIETARY FIBER

Recommendations for adequate intake of dietary fiber during pregnancy are 28 g/day of digestible fiber (IOM 2006) (Table 3.7). In some studies of pregnant women with T1D and GDM, evidence suggests that the second- and third-trimester insulin dosage was correlated negatively with dietary fiber intake, but others found no association (Kitzmiller et al. 2008). Viscous fiber is thought to mitigate postprandial glycemia because of its absorptive properties (McRorie and McKeown 2017). In T2D, this concept was recently supported whether the source of fiber was by supplementation or dietary sources (de Carvalho et al. 2017). In pregnancy, a recent meta-analysis suggested that increased fiber intake alone could influence fetal growth; a low-glycemic-index diet with higher fiber in pregnancy also reduced the risk for macrosomia (Wei et al. 2016). Adequate fiber intake can minimize the risk of, or alleviate, the common pregnancy complaint of constipation, which is the result of slowed digestion. Inclusion of adequate fiber also may increase satiety and aid in the management of appetite. Many pregnant women, including those with diabetes, consume less than the recommended amounts of fiber. When counseling pregnant women to increase fiber, the changes should be made incrementally. A dramatic increase may trigger gastrointestinal discomfort and discourage women from making healthy changes. Pregnant women with diabetes do not need more fiber than women who do not have diabetes, but they should be encouraged to include fiber-rich foods to meet the recommendation. If a food has >5 g dietary fiber, subtract half that amount from the total carbohydrates for insulin bolusing (Wheeler and Pi-Sunyer 2008).

Table 3.7—Selected Food Sources Ranked by Amount of Dietary Fiber and Calories per Standard Food Portion

Food	Standard Portion Size	Calories in Standard Portion	Dietary Fiber in Standard Portion (g)
Beans (navy, pinto, black, kidney, white, great northern, lima), cooked	1/2 cup	104–149	6.2–9.6
Bran, ready-to-eat cereal (100%)	1/3 cup (about 1 ounce)	81	9.1
Split peas, lentils, chickpeas, or cowpeas, cooked	1/2 cup	108–134	5.6–8.1
Artichoke, cooked	1/2 cup hearts	45	7.2
Pear	1 medium	103	5.5
Soybeans, mature, cooked	1/2 cup	149	5.2
Plain rye wafer crackers	2 wafers	73	5.0
Bran, ready-to-eat cereals (various)	1/3–3/4 cup (about 1 oz)	88–91	2.6–5.0
Asian pear	1 small	51	4.4
Green peas, cooked	1/2 cup	59–67	3.5–4.4
Whole-wheat English muffin	1 muffin	134	4.4
Bulgur, cooked	1/2 cup	76	4.1
Mixed vegetables, cooked	1/2 cup	59	4.0
Raspberries	1/2 cup	32	4.0
Sweet potato, baked in skin	1 medium	103	3.8
Blackberries	1/2 cup	31	3.8
Soybeans, green, cooked	1/2 cup	127	3.8
Prunes, stewed	1/2 cup	133	3.8
Shredded wheat, ready-to-eat cereal	1/2 cup (about 1 oz)	95–100	2.7–3.8
Figs, dried	1/4 cup	93	3.7
Apple, with skin	1 small	77	3.6
Pumpkin, canned	1/2 cup	42	3.6
Greens (spinach, collards, turnip greens), cooked	1/2 cup	14–32	2.5–3.5
Almonds	1 ounce	163	3.5
Sauerkraut, canned	1/2 cup	22	3.4
Whole-wheat spaghetti, cooked	1/2 cup	87	3.1
Banana	1 medium	105	3.1
Orange	1 medium	62	3.1

Table 3.7 (continued)

Food	Standard Portion Size	Calories in Standard Portion	Dietary Fiber in Standard Portion (g)
Guava	1 fruit	37	3.0
Potato, baked, with skin	1 small	128	3.0
Oat bran muffin	1 small	178	3.0
Pearled barley, cooked	1/2 cup	97	3.0
Dates	1/4 cup	104	2.9
Winter squash, cooked	1/2 cup	38	2.9
Parsnips, cooked	1/2 cup	55	2.8
Tomato paste	1/4 cup	54	2.7
Broccoli, cooked	1/2 cup	26–27	2.6–2.8
Okra, cooked from frozen	1/2 cup	26	2.6

Source: From U.S. Department of Agriculture, Center for Nutrition Policy and Promotion (2010).

GLYCEMIC INDEX

The glycemic index (GI) is a ranking of foods based on a specific carbohydrate amount and the postprandial incremental glucose response and insulin demand (Brand-Miller and Buyken 2012). This measures quality but not quantity (Augustin et al. 2015). The concept of glycemic load compares the overall effect of a usual portion of food. In practice, the postprandial blood glucose level is measuring the glucose level of an entire meal. A recent meta-analysis of five randomized controlled trials (RCTs) showed that in addition to reducing the need for insulin, a low-GI diet (versus higher-GI diet) in GDM reduced the risk of macrosomia (Wei et al. 2016). Overall, studies in pregnancy suggest a benefit of low-GI diets in GDM on fasting or postprandial glucose and infant birth weight, particularly when fiber intake is increased (Hernandez et al. 2018). GI or glucose level can be used as an additional tool for individuals to improve glucose control based on postprandial results. A glucose level exchange list is available in *Managing Preexisting Diabetes and Pregnancy* (Kitzmiller et al. 2008) and may be useful. More studies are needed in pregnant women with preexisting diabetes.

RESISTANT STARCH AND HIGH-AMYLOSE FOODS

Naturally occurring nondigestible oligosaccharides or foods produced by the modification of starch during processing are termed "resistant starches." Some evidence indicates that these foods may have a beneficial effect on glucose control, but no long-term studies have been conducted on people with diabetes

(Wheeler and Pi-Sunyer 2008, Evert et al. 2014). Food sources include legumes, seeds, whole grains, high-amylose corn, cooked and chilled potatoes, pasta, and rice. Many of these foods are nutrient dense and may be included as healthy carbohydrate choices in the meal plan.

PROTEIN

Additional protein, providing indispensable amino acids, is required during pregnancy for the expansion of maternal plasma volume and amniotic fluid and to support the growth of placental, fetal, and maternal tissue. The RDA for protein in the nonpregnant woman is 0.8 g/kg/day. During the second and third trimester, the requirement increases to 1.1 g/kg/day or an increase of ~25 g/day (IOM 2005, 2006). Protein sources include animal sources (meat, poultry, fish, eggs, milk, cheese, yogurt) and plants, grains, nuts, seeds, and vegetables. Protein has a minimal effect on postprandial glucose excursion and may be useful to provide satiety and necessary calories. Creating a meal plan for a pregnant woman with diabetes who practices a vegan eating style requires skill. Women who have overt nephropathy should meet the 1.1 g/kg RDA for protein, but they should not consume <60 g/day (American Diabetes Association 2018). For example, an 80-kg (176-lb) woman with nephropathy should limit her protein intake to 88 g/day, but a women weighing only 46 kg (101 lb) should meet the minimum recommendation of 60 g/day.

DIETARY FAT

Intake of dietary fat provides energy and essential fatty acids, while enhancing absorption of fat-soluble vitamins. There is no RDA for total dietary fat intake (IOM 2005). Excess fat intake, however, contributes significantly to energy intake. Moreover, it has been shown that it increases insulin resistance in normal pregnancy and is linked to fetal overgrowth in GDM (Sivan et al. 1998, Hernandez et al. 2016). Fats provide more calories per gram than any other calorie source (9 kcal/g), and excess intake may result in excessive weight gain. This may lead to further increased insulin resistance and postpartum weight retention in women with diabetes. It is important to consider the long-term cardiovascular impact of fat intake in pregnant women with diabetes. Meal plans for women with diabetes generally contain 25–40% of daily calories from fat.

Types of fat include saturated (SFA), trans-unsaturated, monounsaturated (MUFA), and polyunsaturated fatty acids (PUFA). In the interest of long-term maternal health, SFA, found primarily in animal products, should be limited to 7–10% of total calories (IOM 2005, U.S Department of Health and Human Services and U.S. Department of Agriculture 2015). *Trans* fat, primarily synthetic, intake should be minimal (IOM 2010). Women with diabetes who have preexisting dyslipidemia should continue to limit their cholesterol intake to <200 mg/day. The remaining 20–30% of daily calories should come from MUFA (e.g., olive oil, avocado, canola oil, almonds) and PUFA (e.g., soybean, corn, and safflower oil).

The adequate intake for essential fatty acids in pregnancy is 13 g/day of omega-6 (n-6) fatty acids and 1.4 g/day of omega-3 (n-3) fatty acids (IOM 2005).

The key omega-3 (n-3) fatty acids include eicosapentaenoic acid and docosahexaenoic acid (DHA). DHA is a PUFA necessary for fetal central nervous system development. DHA is found mainly in cold-water fatty fish, such as salmon. It is recommended that nonpregnant and pregnant women with diabetes eat at least two meals of oily ocean fish per week to reduce the risks of cardiovascular disease and hypertriglyceridemia (American Diabetes Association 2018). In pregnancy, women should avoid eating fish potentially high in mercury and polychlorinated biphenyls. By limiting consumption to 12 oz per week and avoiding consumption of large predatory fish (e.g., swordfish, king mackerel, shark, and tilefish), pregnant women can incorporate seafood in their diet (U.S. Department of Agriculture, Center for Nutrition Policy and Promotions 2012). Information about safe seafood can encourage women with diabetes to include healthy seafood choices in their diet for their long-term health and that of their developing fetus.

MICRONUTRIENTS

SODIUM

The sodium requirement during pregnancy is 2,300 mg/day, the same as for a nonpregnant adult woman without diabetes (IOM 2006). According to the *Dietary Guidelines for Americans, 2010* (U.S. Department of Agriculture, Center for Nutrition Policy and Promotions 2012), "virtually all Americans consume more sodium than they need," and a reduction in salt intake in the U.S. population is recommended (Louie et al. 2011). Pregnant women with diabetes may be encouraged to reduce sodium to recommended levels. According to the *Dietary Guidelines* (U.S. Department of Agriculture, Center for Nutrition Policy and Promotions 2012), some suggestions are as follows:

- Read the nutrition facts label for information on the sodium content of foods and purchase foods that are low in sodium.
- Consume more fresh foods and fewer processed foods that are high in sodium.
- Eat more home-prepared foods, for which you have more control over sodium, and use little or no salt or salt-containing seasonings when cooking or eating foods.
- When eating at restaurants, ask that salt not be added to your food or order lower-sodium options.

FOLATE

Folate functions as a coenzyme in the transfer of single carbon units from one compound to another. A folate deficiency during early gestation is associated with impaired cellular growth and replication resulting in fetal malformations, spontaneous abortions, preterm delivery, and low birth weight (Kitzmiller et al. 2008). As a result of the evidence for the role of folate in the prevention of neural tube defects, the U.S. Public Health Service recommends that all women in the periconceptional period consume 400 µg of folic acid daily from a combination of supplements, fortified foods, and a varied diet. During pregnancy, folate requirements increase to 600 µg/day (IOM 2009). Sources of food folate include oranges and orange juice, beans and peas, and dark green leafy vegetables. Folic acid is added to fortified foods, such as grain and cereal products.

Folate supplementation can mask vitamin B_{12} deficiency in women with T1D who have autoimmune gastritis or malabsorption (American Diabetes Association 2018). Obtaining baseline vitamin B_{12} levels may be useful in these women. Women who follow a vegetarian diet also may need supplementation of vitamin B_{12}.

IRON

The RDA for iron is 27 mg/day throughout pregnancy (IOM 2006). Although iron absorption increases during pregnancy, extra iron is required for fetal erythropoiesis and an increase in maternal red cell mass. Maternal iron deficiency anemia increases the risk of low birth weight, preterm delivery, and perinatal mortality (IOM 2001). Iron supplementation should be initiated if there is laboratory evidence of anemia. In the first and third trimester, this is a hemoglobin of <11.0 g/dL, and in the second trimester it is a hemoglobin of <10.5 g/dL (ACOG 2008, American Diabetes Association 2018). Women with anemia may need elemental iron supplementation of 60–120 mg/day for treatment.

VITAMIN D AND CALCIUM

Vitamin D is necessary to maintain positive calcium homeostasis in pregnancy. A maternal deficiency in vitamin D may lead to low serum calcium in the infant and adversely affect neonatal bone metabolism. Vitamin D is found in egg yolks, fatty fish, and fortified milk. Ready-to-eat breakfast cereals as well as some brands of orange juice, yogurt, margarine, and other food products are now fortified with vitamin D. Current interest and concern surrounding vitamin D intake prompted the IOM to issue the consensus report *Dietary Reference Intakes for Vitamin D and Calcium* in 2010 (IOM 2010). Calcium was included in the report because of its interrelationship with vitamin D. The RDA for vitamin D in pregnancy was set at 600 IU.

Calcium absorption increases in pregnancy. As a result, the RDA for calcium in pregnancy is 1,000 mg/day, the same as for nonpregnant individuals. Adequate calcium intake protects maternal bone mass. Good sources of calcium include milk, yogurt, and cheese. When a pregnant woman with diabetes does not consume adequate calcium from dairy sources, supplementation of 600 mg/day is recommended (IOM 1990).

OTHER NUTRIENTS

Chromium, magnesium, potassium, selenium, and zinc play critical roles in fetal development. Deficiencies in these nutrients also may affect carbohydrate tolerance (Kitzmiller et al. 2008). Currently, no evidence supports a recommendation to routinely supplement pregnant women with diabetes with the antioxidants vitamin C and vitamin E beyond the IOM recommendations for all pregnant women. It is important to counsel pregnant women with diabetes to eat healthful, nutrient-dense diets to achieve the DRIs for adequacy (see Table 3.2). An extensive review of specific nutrients is available in *Management of Preexisiting Diabetes and Pregnancy* (Kitzmiller et al. 2008).

VITAMIN AND MINERAL SUPPLEMENTATION

Multivitamin and mineral supplements are recommended for women who have poor diets, have iron deficiency anemia, and include little or no animal protein in their diets. Women with multiple pregnancies, with other high-risk conditions, and who use tobacco or abuse alcohol or drugs also should take a supplement. Pregnant women with diabetes may need to take supplements to meet the recommended levels of vitamins, minerals, and trace elements. Nutrient-dense food choices should be encouraged in all pregnant women with diabetes (Hernandez et al. 2018).

FOOD SAFETY

CAFFEINE

High caffeine intake during pregnancy is associated with spontaneous miscarriage and low birth weight, but it has not been shown to correlate with birth defects. Reports have shown that large quantities of caffeine ingested (>300 mg/day) increase the risk of intrauterine growth restriction and spontaneous abortion (Higdon and Frei 2006). Pregnant women who consume caffeine-containing beverages should do so in moderation. The suggested limit is ≤300 mg caffeine daily (Table 3.8).

Table 3.8—Caffeine Content of Common Beverages

Beverage		Serving Size	Caffeine (mg/serving)
Coffee	brewed	8 oz	72
	instant	8 oz	64
	epresso	4 oz	256
Tea	black	8 oz	48
	green	8 oz	40
Energy drink		16 oz	48-560
Cola		12 oz	48
Energy shot		2 oz	*

Source: Adapted from U.S. Department of Health and Human Services and U.S. Department of Agriculture (2015).

*Some dietary supplements and energy shots contain caffeine, but their caffeine content is not required to be listed on nutrition labeling.

ALCOHOL

Alcohol should not be consumed by pregnant women, including those with diabetes (IOM 2006).

NONNUTRITIVE SWEETENERS

Use of nonnutritive sweeteners classified as Generally Recognized as Safe is acceptable in moderation during pregnancy. These include acesulfame potassium, aspartame, saccharin, stevia, sucralose, and neotame (American Dietetic Association [now Academy of Nutrition and Dietetics] 2008). Blends of artificial sweeteners that contain dextrose should be counted as carbohydrate in the meal plan.

HERBAL MEDICINES AND SUPPLEMENTS

Popular culture views herbal, "natural," botanical, or other supplements as safe. Different cultures may include use of these teas and other herbals routinely. Heath professionals should ask pregnant women with diabetes whether they use any of these substances so they may be evaluated for potential risk during pregnancy, including effects on blood glucose control (American Dietetic Association [now Academy of Nutrition and Dietetics] 2008).

LISTERIA

Women with diabetes are at risk for foodborne illness. Pregnant women are at high risk to become sick from listeria, a bacteria found in some foods. Infection can result in miscarriage, stillbirth, preterm delivery, or neonatal illness (U.S. Department of Agriculture, Food Safety 2011). To avoid infection, pregnant women should not consume the following:

- Hot dogs, luncheon meats, or other deli meats unless they are reheated until steaming hot.
- Soft cheese such as feta, queso blanco, queso fresco, Brie, Camembert, blue-veined cheeses, and Panela unless it is labeled as made with pasteurized milk.
- Salads made in the store, such as ham salad, egg salad, chicken salad, tuna salad, or seafood salad.
- Raw or unpasteurized milk.
- Refrigerated paté, meat spreads, or smoked seafood (unless cooked). Shelf-stable or canned paté or meat spreads can be consumed.

MERCURY

Women should follow the *Dietary Guidelines 2010* (U.S. Department of Agriculture, Center for Nutrition Policy and Promotion 2012) for inclusion of safe seafood as outlined in the section "Dietary Fat."

EXERCISE AS A TREATMENT MODALITY

Pregnancy is an insulin-resistant state. Cardiovascular conditioning exercise facilitates glucose utilization among other things by increasing insulin binding to and affinity for its receptor and receptor number (Pederson et al. 1980). In this way, exercise can reduce peripheral resistance to insulin and should reduce the need for insulin administration in pregnancy in both GDM and preexisting diabetes.

Exercise during pregnancy is widely accepted as safe (ACOG 2015a). Women may be taught to palpate their own uterus during exercise and stop the exercise if they detect a contraction. In addition to proper frequency, intensity, duration, and modality of exercise, self-monitoring of uterine activity may provide a means of surveillance that allows for the safe prescription of exercise during the third trimester. Although exercise during pregnancy in women with diabetes should be encouraged, pregnant women should not engage in contact sports, such as hockey, football, or soccer, where injury is likely, or in activities with a high potential for falling, such as downhill skiing or gymnastics. Typically, any low-impact exercise at room temperature is encouraged, including walking, yoga, or stationary biking.

Specifically for GDM, exercise may be used to reduce GDM risk and as part of lifestyle modification to reduce the chance of needing insulin after GDM diagnosis. The effects of exercise on glucose metabolism can become apparent after 4 weeks of training and affect both hepatic glucose output (reflected by fasting glucose levels) and glucose utilization (reflected by glucose values after a 50-g oral glucose challenge) (Jovanovic-Peterson et al. 1989). When exercise is used to help manage glucose in GDM, upper-body cardiovascular training has resulted in lower levels of glycemia than in women treated by diet only (Jovanovic-Peterson et al. 1989, Durak et al. 1990).

SELECTED READINGS

Academy of Nutrition and Dietetics (formerly American Dietetic Association). *Medical Nutrition Therapy, Evidence-Based Guides for Practice: Type 1 & 2 Diabetes Mellitus Evidence-Based Guide for Practice.* Chicago, American Dietetic Association, 2008

American Diabetes Association. Nutrition recommendations and interventions for diabetes. Position statement. *Diabetes Care* 2008;31(Suppl. 1):S61–S68

California Department of Public Health. Prenatal weight gain grids. Available from www.cdph.ca.gov/pubsforms/forms/Pages/MaternalandChildHealth.aspx. Accessed 8 September 2012

California Diabetes and Pregnancy Program. *Sweet Success California Diabetes and Pregnancy Program Guidelines for Care.* Revised ed. Sacramento, CA, State of California Department of Public Health, Maternal, Child and Adolescent Health Division, 2008

Lawrence RA, Lawrence RM. *Breastfeeding: A Guide for the Medical Profession.* 7th ed. Philadelphia, PA, Elsevier Mosby, 2011

Thomas A. Pregnancy with pre-existing diabetes. In *The Art and Science of Diabetes Self-Management Education. A Desk Reference for Healthcare Professionals.* Messing C, Ed. Chicago, IL, American Association of Diabetes Educators, 2006

REFERENCES

Academy of Nutrition and Dietetics (formerly American Dietetic Association). *Medical Nutrition Therapy, Evidence-Based Guides for Practice: Gestational Diabetes Mellitus Evidence-Based Guide for Practice.* Chicago, American Dietetic Association, 2017. Available from www.andeal.org

American College of Obstetricians and Gynecologists. Practice bulletin no. 95: Anemia in pregnancy. *Obstet Gynecol* 2008;112:201–207

American College of Obstetricians and Gynecologists. Committee opinion no. 650: Physical activity and exercise during pregnancy and the postpartum period. *Obstet Gynecol* 2015a;126(6):e135–e142

American College of Obstetricians and Gynecologists. Practice bulletin no. 156: Obesity in pregnancy. *Obstet Gynecol* 2015b;126(6):112–126

American Diabetes Association. Standards of medical care in diabetes, 2018. *Diabetes Care* 2018;41(Suppl. 1):S137–S143

American Dietetic Association (now Academy of Nutrition and Dietetics). Nutrition and lifestyle for a healthy pregnancy outcome. Position statement. *J Am Diet Assoc* 2008;108:553–560

Augustin LS, Kendall CW, Jenkins DJ, Willett WC, Astrup A, Barclay AW, et al. Glycemic index, glycemic load and glycemic response: an International Scientific Consensus Summit from the International Carbohydrate Quality Consortium (ICQC). *Nutr Metab Cardiovasc Dis* 2015;25(9):795–815

Barbour LA, Hernandez TL. Maternal non-glycemic contributors to fetal growth in obesity and gestational diabetes: spotlight on lipids. *Curr Diab Rep* 2018; 18(6):37

Brand-Miller JC, Buyken AE. The glycemic index issue. *Curr Opin Lipidol* 2012;23(1):62–67

Buschur EO, Stetson B, Barbour LA, Thung S, ed. *Diabetes in Pregnancy.* EndoText.org, 2018

Catalano PM, Mele L, Landon MB, Ramin SM, Reddy UM, Casey B, et al. Inadequate weight gain in overweight and obese pregnant women: what is the effect on fetal growth? *Am J Obstet Gynecol* 2014;211(2):137.e1–e7

Centers for Disease Control and Prevention. Adult BMI calculator. Updated October 31, 2018. Available from www.cdc.gov/healthyweight/assessing/bmi/adult_bmi/english_bmi_calculator/bmi_calculator.html. Accessed on 22 February 2019

de Carvalho CM, de Paula TP, Viana LV, Machado VM, de Almeida JC, Azevedo MJ. Plasma glucose and insulin responses after consumption of breakfasts with different sources of soluble fiber in type 2 diabetes patients: a randomized crossover clinical trial. *Am J Clin Nutr* 2017;106:1238–1245

Dennedy MC, Avalos G, O'Reilly MW, O'Sullivan EP, Gaffney G, Dunne F. Atlantic-DIP: raised maternal body mass index (BMI) adversely affects maternal and fetal outcomes in glucose-tolerant women according to the International Association of Diabetes and Pregnancy Study Group. *J Clin Endocrin Metab* 2012;97:E608–E612

Deputy NP, Dub B, Sharma AJ. Prevalence and trends in prepregnancy normal weight - 48 states, New York City, and District of Columbia, 2011–2015. *Morb Mortal Wkly Rep* 2018;66(5152):1402–1407

Dornhurst A, Nicholls JSD, Probst F, Patterson CM, Hollier KL, Elkeles RS, Beard RW. Calorie restriction for the treatment of gestational diabetes. *Diabetes* 1991;40:161–164

Durak EP, Jovanovic-Peterson L, Peterson CM. Physical and glycemic responses of women with gestational diabetes to a moderately intense exercise program. *Diabetes Educ* 1990;16(4):309–312

Evert AB, Boucher JL, Cypress M, Dunbar SA, Franz MJ, Mayer-Davis EJ, et al. Nutrition therapy recommendations for the management of adults with diabetes. *Diabetes Care* 2014;37(Suppl.):S120–S143

Flegal KM, Kruszon-Moran D, Carroll MD, Fryar CD, Ogden CL. Trends in obesity among adults in the United States, 2005 to 2014. *JAMA* 2016;315(21):2284–2291

Hernandez TL, Mande A, Barbour LA. Nutrition therapy within and beyond gestational diabetes. *Diab Res Clin Pract* 2018;145:39–50

Hernandez TL, van Pelt RE, Anderson MA, Reece MS, Reynolds RM, de la Houssaye BA, et al. Women with gestational diabetes mellitus randomized to a higher-complex carbohydrate/low-fat diet manifest lower adipose tissue insulin resistance, inflammation, glucose, and free fatty acids: a pilot study. *Diabetes Care* 2016;39(1):39–42

Higdon JV, Frei B. Coffee and health: a review of recent human research. *Crit Rev Food Sci Nutr* 2006;46:101–123

Holme AM, Roland MC, Lorentzen B, Michelsen TM, Henriksen T. Placental glucose transfer: a human in vivo study. *PLoS One* 2015;10:e0117084

Institute of Medicine. *Dietary Reference Intakes for Energy, Carbohydrate, Fiber, Fat, Fatty Acids, Cholesterol, Protein, and Amino Acids.* Washington, DC, The National Academies Press, 2005

Institute of Medicine, Food and Nutrition Board. *National Academy of Sciences (US). Nutrition During Pregnancy: Weight Gain and Nutrient Supplements. Report of the Committee on Nutritional Status During Pregnancy and Lactation.* Washington, DC, The National Academies Press, 1990

Institute of Medicine, Food and Nutrition Board. *Dietary Reference Intakes for Vitamin A, Vitamin K, Arsenic, Boron, Chromium, Copper, Iodine, Iron, Manganese,*

Molybdenum, Nickel, Silicon, Vanadium and Zinc. Washington, DC, The National Academies Press, 2001

Institute of Medicine, Food and Nutrition Board. *Dietary Reference Intakes: The Essential Guide to Nutrient Requirements.* Washington, DC, The National Academies Press, 2006

Institute of Medicine, Food and Nutrition Board. *Dietary Reference Intakes for Calcium and Vitamin D.* Washington, DC, The National Academies Press, 2010

Institute of Medicine, National Research Council. *Weight Gain During Pregnancy: Reexamining the Guidelines.* Rasmussen KM, Taktine AL, Eds. Washington, DC, The National Academies Press, 2009

Johnstone FD, Lindsay RS, Steel J. Type 1 diabetes and pregnancy: trends in birth weight over 40 years at a single clinic. *Obstet Gynec* 2006;107:1297–1302

Jovanovic L, Knopp RH, Kim H, Cefalu WT, Zhu X-D, Lee YJ, Simpson JL, Mills JL. For the Diabetes in Early Pregnancy Study Group: elevated pregnancy losses at high and low extremes of maternal glucose in early normal and diabetic pregnancy. Evidence for a protective adaptation in diabetes. *Diabetes Care* 2005;28:1113–1117

Jovanovic-Peterson L, Durak EP, Peterson CM. Randomized trial of diet versus diet plus cardiovascular conditioning on glucose levels in gestational diabetes. *Am J Obstet Gynecol* 1989;161(2):415–419

Kitzmiller JL, Jovanovic L, Brown FM, Coustan DR, Reader DM (Eds.). *Managing Preexisting Diabetes and Pregnancy: Technical Reviews and Consensus Recommendations for Care.* Alexandria, VA, American Diabetes Association, 2008

Knopp RH, Magee MS, Raisys V, Benedetti TJ. Metabolic effects of hypocaloric diets in management of gestational diabetes. *Diabetes* 1991;40:165–171

Louie JCY, Markovic TP, Perera N, Foote P, Foote D, Petocz P, Ross JC, Brand-Miller JC. A randomized controlled trial investigating the effects of a low-glycemic index diet on pregnancy outcomes in gestational diabetes mellitus. *Diabetes Care* 2011;34:2341–2346

McRorie JW, Jr., McKeown NM. Understanding the physics of functional fibers in the gastrointestinal tract: an evidence-based approach to resolving enduring misconceptions about insoluble and soluble fiber. *J Acad Nutr Diet* 2017; 117:251–264

Nicklas JM, Barbour LA. Optimizing weight for maternal and infant health—tenable, or too late? *Expert Rev Endocrinol Metab* 2015;10(2):227–242

Pedersen O, Beck-Nielsen H, Heding L. Increased insulin receptors after exercise in patients with insulin-dependent diabetes mellitus. *N Engl J Med* 1980;302(16):886–892

Reader D, Splett P, Gunderson E. Impact of gestational diabetes mellitus nutrition practice guidelines implemented by registered dietitians on pregnancy outcome. *J Am Diet Assoc* 2006;106:1426–1433

Rizzo T, Metzger BE, Burns WJ, Burns K. Correlations between antepartum maternal metabolism and intelligence of offspring. *N Engl J Med* 1991;325(13):911–916

Sivan E, Homko CJ, Whittaker PG, Reece EA, Chen X, Boden G. Free fatty acids and insulin resistance during pregnancy. *J Clin Endocrinol Metab* 1998;83(7): 2338–2342

U.S. Department of Agriculture, Center for Nutrition Policy and Promotion. Report of the Dietary Guidelines Advisory Committee on the Dietary Guidelines for Americans, 2010. Available from www.fns.usda.gov/dietaryguidelines. Accessed 10 August 2012

U.S. Department of Agriculture, Center for Nutrition Policy and Promotion. My plate daily meal plans for pregnancy and breastfeeding. Available from www.choosemyplate.gov/mypyramidmoms. Accessed 8 September 2012

U.S. Department of Agriculture, Food Safety. Food safety for pregnant women, 2006 (slightly revised 2011). Available from www.fda.gov/Food/ResourcesForYou/Consumers/SelectedHealthTopics/ucm312704.htm. Accessed 28 August 2012

U.S. Department of Health and Human Services and U.S. Department of Agriculture, 2015–2020. *Dietary Guidelines for Americans.* 8th ed. Washington, DC, U.S. Department of Health and Human Services, 2015

Wahabi HA, Esmaeil SA, Fayed A, Al-Shaikh G, Alzeidan RA. Pre-existing diabetes mellitus and adverse pregnancy outcomes. *BMC Res Notes* 2012;5:496

Wei J, Heng W, Gao J. Effects of low glycemic index diets on gestational diabetes mellitus: a meta-analysis of randomized controlled clinical trials. *Medicine (Baltimore)* 2016;95:e3792

Wheeler ML, Pi-Sunyer FX. Carbohydrate issues: type and amount. *J Am Diet Assoc* 2008;108:S34–S39

Xu Z, Wen Z, Zhou Y, Li D, Luo Z. Inadequate weight gain in obese women and the risk of small for gestational age (SGA): a systematic review and meta-analysis. *J Matern Fetal Neonatal Med* 2017;30(3):357–367

Medication Management of Diabetes in Pregnancy

Highlights
Medication Management of Diabetes in Pregnancy

■ In women with preexisting diabetes who require medications to achieve goals, insulin requirements often reach a nadir at the end of the first trimester.

■ Insulin is the mainstay of medical management in preexisting diabetes and gestational diabetes mellitus (GDM) during pregnancy for those who require medication to achieve goals. Premixed insulins usually are avoided in pregnancy because the long- and short-acting insulin doses cannot be adjusted independently to optimize glucose control.

■ Insulin pumps can be used in pregnancy with good results.

■ If an oral agent is used to manage GDM, metformin is associated with lower rates of macrosomia and neonatal hypoglycemia compared to glyburide, but it fails to achieve adequate glucose control in roughly half of the women requiring medication for GDM. Both oral agents cross the placenta.

Medication Management of Diabetes in Pregnancy

Medication management of diabetes during pregnancy differs in important ways compared to the nonpregnant state. The most obvious difference is that hyperglycemia exerts potentially devastating effects on the fetus throughout pregnancy with a risk of congenital defects of ~25% if hemoglobin A_{1c} (A1C) is >10% during organogenesis (American College of Obstetricians and Gynecologists [ACOG] 2005). An elevated risk to the offspring persists throughout pregnancy and beyond with a higher likelihood of macrosomia, preterm birth, respiratory distress, and development of obesity and type 2 diabetes (T2D) later in life (National Institute for Health and Clinical Excellence 2008, ACOG 2013). A more subtle, but equally important, difference in diabetes management during pregnancy is that evolving metabolic changes are occurring to meet maternal needs and provide fuel for the growing fetoplacental unit (Freinkel 1980). Embedding diabetes management strategies in a firm understanding of the metabolic changes that occur in pregnancy is essential to achieving glycemic control.

METABOLIC CHANGES DURING PREGNANCY

Women with type 1 diabetes (T1D) may note that blood glucose control during the first trimester is more unstable than usual and severe hypoglycemia is more common (Evers et al. 2002, Garcia-Patterson et al. 2010). This occurs because of transfer of glucose and gluconeogenic substrate to the fetus. By 12 weeks of gestation, insulin requirements in women with T1D often diminish by 10–20% compared to the dose before conception (Garcia-Patterson et al. 2010) (Figure 4.1).

The diabetogenic stress of pregnancy typically ensues in the mid-trimester and daily insulin requirements begin to rise (Garcia-Patterson et al. 2010). At this time, the mother switches from a primarily glucose-based to a lipid-based energy economy derived from either circulating fats or stored adipose tissue to spare glucose for fetal growth. Throughout the second and third trimesters, insulin requirements gradually increase to as much as twice the total daily dosage of insulin needed before pregnancy. Pregnant women with normal physiology are able to overcome this mounting insulin resistance by increasing insulin production to maintain normal glucose levels. When endogenous insulin production fails to increase, however, this reflects an evolving disease process in women with preexisting diabetes or results in a new diagnosis of gestational diabetes mellitus (GDM).

By the third trimester, basal insulin levels are higher than normal nongravid levels and eating produces a two- to threefold greater outpouring of insulin. These

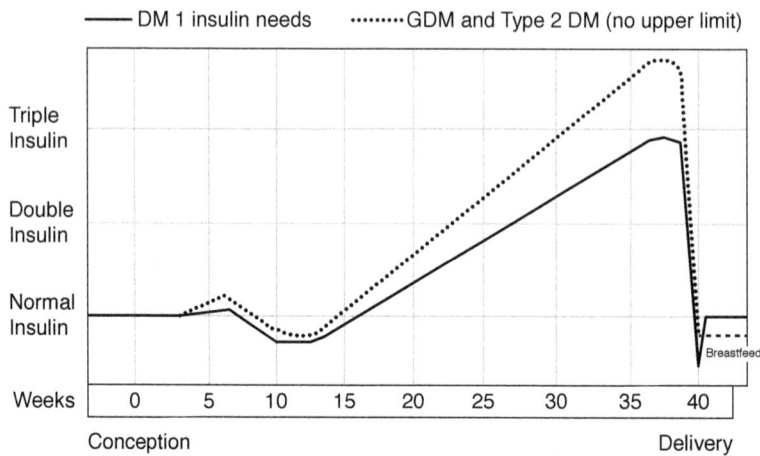

Figure 4.1—Insulin requirements during pregnancy.
Source: Shields and Tsay (2015). © CDPH 2012; Funded by Federal Title V Block Grant through the Maternal, Child and Adolescent Health Division.

increases in plasma insulin are opposed by diminished responsiveness to insulin action because of increased maternal production of cortisol and placental production of contra-insulin hormones, such as human placental lactogen, estrogen, and progesterone. Placental growth and production of these contra-insulin hormones plateau at ~36 weeks. As a result, the dosage of insulin necessary to maintain euglycemia peaks at 37 weeks (Garcia-Patterson et al. 2010).

After delivery of the placenta, human placental lactogen, estrogen, and progesterone rapidly clear from the circulation, leading to a marked decrease in insulin resistance. The dosage of insulin required postpartum often drops by 50% in women with preexisting diabetes and must be recalculated based on postpartum weight, diet, exercise, and plans for breast-feeding. For women with GDM, medication may be discontinued immediately after delivery.

Although comprehensive treatment of diabetes during pregnancy includes dietary control, exercise, glucose monitoring, and medication management (Hartling et al. 2013, Crowther et al. 2005), the remainder of this chapter will focus exclusively on medication management.

ANTENATAL INSULIN USE

Insulin has the longest track record with regard to medication management of diabetes during pregnancy and is generally considered the first-line agent by the American College of Obstetricians and Gynecologists (2018) and the American Diabetes Association (2018). Human insulins are the least immunogenic of all insulins, but insulin analogs tend to provide better glycemic control and patient satisfaction (Hirsch 2005). A recent retrospective population-based cohort study showed first-trimester exposure to insulin analogs (lispro, aspart glulisine, detemir, glargine) did not increase the risk of major congenital anomalies, compared with human insulin, and possibly had a lower risk of congenital heart defects (Wang et al. 2018).

The primary goal of insulin replacement is to achieve plasma glucose concentrations nearly identical to those observed in pregnant women without diabetes, but this must be balanced against the risk of hypoglycemia. The optimum insulin injection schedule for women with preexisting diabetes during pregnancy has not been established, and many insulin regimens can be used to achieve glycemic control (O'Neill et al. 2017). Insulin administration normally includes both a basal stage, to prevent hepatic gluconeogenesis and mobilization of free fatty acids from adipose tissue, and a meal stage to cover dietary carbohydrate intake.

Basal insulin is required without regard for meals or physical activity. Any glucose regimen should address basal insulin requirements through intermediate- or long-acting insulin that is dosed every 12–24 h. The basal requirement in pregnancy is typically met with twice-daily injection of intermediate-acting NPH (neutral protamine Hagedorn) insulin or a daily or twice-daily injection of a long-acting insulin analog. There are an ever-growing number of basal insulin analogs, including insulin glargine (Lantus, Sanofi Aventis), insulin detemir (Levemir, Novo Nordisk), and the newest one to market, insulin degludec (Tresiba, Novo Nordisk). Recently, the U.S. Food and Drug Administration (FDA) changed the classification of insulin detemir to pregnancy category B based on the results of a multinational, randomized controlled trial (RCT) of 310 pregnant women with T1D that showed no difference in the incidence of adverse maternal or fetal outcomes in women using insulin detemir compared with women using NPH (Mathiesen et al. 2012). Two noninferiority trials suggested that detemir is not inferior to NPH in women with T1D (Mathiesen et al. 2012), T2D, and GDM (Herrera et al. 2015), and an RCT of women with T1D showed similar perinatal outcomes (Hod et al. 2014). Insulin glargine is an FDA pregnancy category C drug. Studies outside of pregnancy suggest glargine use is associated with decreased fasting blood glucose, decreased A1C, and decreased nocturnal hypoglycemia compared to NPH; however, the efficacy and safety data in pregnancy are not robust. With regard to insulin degludec, there is extremely limited pregnancy data, but a case series suggested no currently identified risks (Bonora et al. 2019). On the basis of currently available data, intermediate- or long-acting insulins are reasonable options during pregnancy.

The meal stage of insulin secretion is addressed with a short-acting insulin analog, such as insulin lispro or insulin aspart. Both are FDA pregnancy category B drugs and are considered safe to use during pregnancy (Mathiesen et al. 2012). Like long-acting insulin analogs, more short-acting analogs enter the market regularly, but this review is limited to those that are most commonly used in pregnancy. Recently glulisine was introduced but data in pregnancy are limited. Regular insulin generally should be avoided for mealtime coverage because it must be administered 30–60 min before a meal, the peak effect occurs 2–5 h later, and it lasts for 5–8 h (Table 4.1). Shorter-acting insulin analogs, such as lispro or aspart, have quicker absorption, and thus patients may take insulin immediately before eating each meal.

Given the evolving insulin requirements during pregnancy, the combination of basal and mealtime coverage permits frequent dose adjustments to achieve glycemic control. Premixed insulins should be avoided during pregnancy because

Table 4.1—Onset, Peak, and Duration of Insulins Commonly Used in Pregnancy

Insulin	Onset of Action (min)	Time to Peak Concentration (min)	Maximum Duration of Action (h)
Short acting			
Regular insulin	30–60	90–120	5–12
Insulin lispro	10–15	30–80	3–4
Insulin aspart	10–15	40–50	3–5
Insulin glulisine	10–15	55	3–5
Long acting			
NPH insulin	60–120	240–280	16–18
Insulin glargine	60–120	None	24
Insulin detemir	60–120	None	20

NPH, neutral protamine Hagedorn.

Source: Adapted from Trujillo (2007).

the doses cannot be adjusted independently. Table 4.2 shows a suggested calculation to determine a starting dose of insulin for women with preexisting diabetes or for women with GDM who have consistently elevated blood glucose who are insulin-naïve. The total amount of insulin can then be divided during the day using the proportions detailed in Figure 4.2. Note that Figure 4.2, however, is just a starting place and providers must work with patients to adjust this regimen to fit the patient's lifestyle and glucose values. Furthermore, with the increasing acceptability of long-acting insulin, particularly detemir, which is an FDA category B drug, pregnancy insulin algorithms increasingly include detemir rather than NPH. When detemir is used, it is commonly given either once or twice per day and cannot be mixed with rapid-acting insulin. The total insulin amount needed can still be calculated, but 40% is given using long-acting insulin and 60% using rapid-acting insulin (20% at each meal if carbohydrate amount is similar at all meals).

Table 4.2—Worksheet to Calculate Insulin Total Daily Dose for Insulin-Naïve Women

1. Patient's current weight in kg =_____
2. Insulin dose by pregnancy trimester
   First→0.8 units/kg
   Second→1.0 units/kg
   Third→1.2 units/kg
3. Total Daily Dose (TDD) = weight in kg (#1) × desired units/kg of insulin (#2)
4. Consider decreasing the TDD by 25% when initiating insulin as an outpatient or in an insulin-naïve patient.

Source: Adapted from Blum (2016).

Insulin dosing regimen

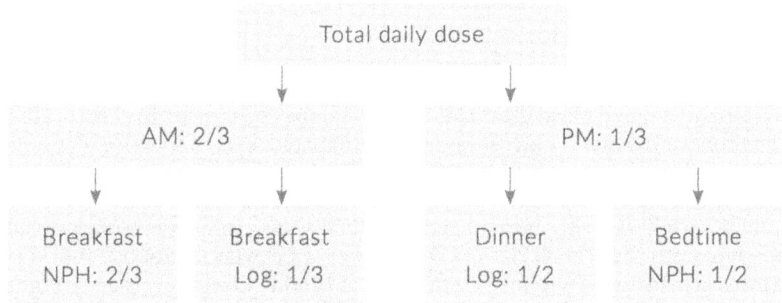

Figure 4.2—Proposed insulin dosing regimen.

INSULIN PUMPS

Because the ultimate goal of glycemic control is to mimic normal pancreatic insulin release, some clinicians prefer continuous subcutaneous insulin infusion (CSII) through an insulin pump. Insulin pumps deliver a basal rate of rapid-acting insulin with pulse-dose increments before meals based on premeal glucose values and anticipated intake of carbohydrate. They have been used safely and successfully during pregnancy. Many women prefer an insulin pump as it may provide more flexibility in timing and composition of meals. Two meta-analyses of RCTs comparing women treated with multiple daily injections to women treated with CSII showed no significant difference in pregnancy outcomes or glycemic control (Mukhopadhyay et al. 2007, Ranasinghe et al. 2015).

In pregnancy, the basal infusion rate is usually <50% of the total daily dose of insulin. Many women will require at least three infusion rates throughout the day, for example, midnight to 4:00 A.M., 4:00 A.M. to 10:00 A.M., 10:00 A.M. to midnight. The lowest basal dose is usually administered from midnight to 4:00 A.M. to help prevent nocturnal hypoglycemia. Between 4:00 A.M. and 10:00 A.M., in response to earlier increased secretion of cortisol and growth hormone level, the basal rate of insulin must be increased. The progressive increase in contra-insulin hormones accompanying pregnancy will require a corresponding increase in basal infusion rates, meal boluses, and insulin sensitivity factor. If the basal infusion rates are calculated properly, glucose concentrations will be within target before meals, and each meal or snack will require a bolus of insulin. The remaining >50% of the total daily dose of insulin is given as meal boluses. Fixed boluses may be used with 30% given at breakfast, 25% at lunch, 25% at dinner, and the remaining 15–20% given with snacks. Alternately, a woman can use a carbohydrate ratio, in which the pump is programmed to give 1 unit of insulin for a given amount of carbohydrates (e.g., 1 unit of insulin given for every 8 g of carbohydrate). This carbohydrate ratio may differ with the time of day. The disadvantages of insulin pump therapy are the cost of an insulin pump and supplies, and the potential for hyperglycemia and diabetic ketoacidosis to develop rapidly if there is pump failure. Sensors and closed-loop pumps are increasingly used in pregnancy, although outcome data are limited.

DOSAGE ADJUSTMENT

Patients must frequently perform blood glucose monitoring and learn to anticipate insulin needs based on the carbohydrate content of the upcoming meal, the preprandial blood glucose, and the anticipated level of exercise. Patients are encouraged to check blood glucose levels frequently, although the optimal frequency of testing has not been determined (ACOG 2018). There is evidence that women with T1D who use continuous glucose monitoring have improved neonatal outcomes (Feig et al. 2017). Women with T1D who do not use continuous glucose monitoring often need to check their blood glucose levels up to eight times daily (before and after each meal, at bedtime, and in the middle of the night). Correction dosing can be continued in pregnancy, but the goal should be to prevent hyperglycemia proactively rather than manage it after it occurs. In women with T2D or GDM, it is reasonable to measure blood glucose levels four times daily (fasting and 1 or 2 h after each meal). Blood glucose also should be tested with any symptoms of hypoglycemia and before driving a vehicle.

Results should be recorded in a form that permits recognition of glycemic patterns. This can be done with a paper log or an electronic application. The essential principles for any successful insulin regimen include observation of glucose patterns and gradual (usually 10–20%) dose adjustments.

Dosage adjustments require looking at the complete clinical picture, including whether patients are taking the medications as prescribed, extenuating life circumstances that make glycemic control difficult (e.g., working nights or having minimal flexibility at work), exercise, and dietary patterns (e.g., sugary beverages). For example, a patient experiencing elevated fasting blood glucose upon waking should have her evening or before-bed intermediate- or long-acting insulin up-titrated. Elevated preprandial blood glucose levels can typically be addressed by up-titrating the morning intermediate- or long-acting insulin. Depending on the clinical scenario and distribution of elevated values throughout the day, postprandial blood glucose can be addressed by evaluating dietary intake and up-titrating mealtime or morning basal insulin.

HYPOGLYCEMIA

Episodes of hypoglycemia (blood glucose <70 mg/dL) warrant close attention. All patients should be counseled regarding signs and symptoms of hypoglycemia (increased heart rate, sweating, tremors, hunger, tingling, confusion, irritability, seizure) and what to do in response. Recommended algorithms include taking four glucose tablets or 1/2 cup of juice and rechecking the blood glucose in 15 min. Patients prescribed insulin also should be prescribed glucagon with training for a family member in how to respond to hypoglycemia if the patient is unresponsive or uncooperative.

INSULIN USE AND PRETERM DELIVERY

Preterm delivery can be particularly hazardous and presents a special therapeutic dilemma in pregnant women with diabetes. Sympathomimetics, such as terbutaline and ritodrine, are capable of causing rapid and extreme elevations in maternal glucose concentration and possibly ketoacidosis and should be avoided in women with diabetes. Magnesium sulfate is prescribed just before birth to patients expected to deliver before 32 weeks of gestation to lessen the likelihood of cerebral palsy in the premature neonate. Indomethacin or calcium channel blockers may be used for tocolysis in women with diabetes. Tocolytic therapy should be undertaken only in centers in which continuous, experienced maternal–fetal supervision is available. Throughout parenteral tocolytic therapy, maternal glucose levels initially should be measured hourly and every 2–4 h once blood glucose is stable. Intravenous (IV) insulin should be administered as necessary.

Corticosteroids, used to accelerate fetal lung maturation in anticipated preterm delivery, can further exacerbate hyperglycemia. The usual dose of corticosteroids is two doses of betamethasone 12 mg given intramuscularly (IM) 24 h apart or four doses of dexamethasone 6 mg given IM 12 h apart. Blood glucose concentrations should be checked frequently, and supplemental rapid-acting insulin should be given as needed or short-acting insulin given as a continuous IV infusion during corticosteroid administration and for several days afterward.

INSULIN USE DURING LABOR AND DELIVERY

Intrapartum glycemic control plays a major role in the well-being of the neonate. Maternal hyperglycemia during labor may be associated with fetal acidemia and is a major cause of neonatal hypoglycemia. At the onset of active labor, insulin requirements decrease, and glucose requirements are relatively constant at ~2.5 mg/kg/min (1.1 mg/lb/min) (Jovanovic 2004). The goal is to maintain a plasma glucose concentration between 70 mg/dL and 110 mg/dL. An insulin drip is advisable for any blood glucose during labor >120 mg/dL to maintain plasma glucose concentration in the desired range and reduce the risk of neonatal hypoglycemia. A woman with an insulin pump may be allowed to continue her pump during labor, adjusting basal rates as needed, although, in our clinical practice, we typically discontinue the pump and utilize an IV insulin drip. Potential management algorithms for planned induction and cesarean section are provided in Tables 4.3 and 4.4.

Table 4.3—Management for Planned Induction of Labor

■ On the evening before elective induction, the usual bedtime dose of intermediate-acting insulin may be given.
■ On the morning of induction, insulin is withheld and an IV infusion of normal saline or 5% dextrose in half-normal saline at 100–125 mL/h (to provide for energy requirements) is begun.
■ Once active labor commences or plasma glucose level falls to <70 mg/dL (<3.9 mmol/L), normal saline should be changed to 5% dextrose in half-normal saline, and infused at a rate of 100–125 mL/min.
■ Glucose level should be monitored hourly, and if it is <60 mg/dL (<3.3 mmol/L), the infusion rate of dextrose-containing fluid should be doubled for the subsequent hour.
■ If the plasma glucose concentration rises to >120 mg/dL (>6.7 mmol/L), an infusion of short-acting insulin in normal saline should be added by piggyback into the dextrose-containing IV. The concentration of insulin in the normal saline can be varied to avoid fluid overload. An example of the starting point would be 25 units of insulin in 250 mL of saline with an infusion rate of 10 mL/h through an infusion pump.

Table 4.4 — Management for Planned Elective Cesarean Delivery

- The bedtime dose of intermediate-acting insulin may be given the night before surgery, and surgery should be scheduled for early morning.
- The woman is instructed to take nothing by mouth (NPO) after midnight, and the morning insulin is not given the day of surgery.
- If surgery is later in the day, one-third to one-half of the woman's intermediate-acting dose of insulin may be given on the morning of surgery and every 8 h if surgery is delayed.
- A dextrose infusion as described previously may be started if the glucose concentration falls to <60 mg/dL (<3.3 mmol/L).
- Alternatively, glycemic control before elective cesarean delivery can be achieved with an infusion of 1–2 units/h IV regular insulin given simultaneously with 5 g/h dextrose. The insulin infusion should be discontinued immediately before surgery.
- Hourly blood glucose determinations are recommended to allow for individualization of these protocols.

ORAL ANTIDIABETIC AGENTS FOR WOMEN WITH GDM

Although insulin has long been the standard for management of diabetes in pregnancy, the Society for Maternal Fetal Medicine (2018), National Institute for Health and Care Excellence (2015), and the International Federation of Gynecology and Obstetrics (Hod et al. 2015) all accept oral antidiabetic agents as first-line therapy for women with GDM. The only oral diabetes medications widely used in pregnancy are glyburide and metformin. Note, however, that neither medication is FDA approved for use in pregnancy.

METFORMIN

Metformin is an oral biguanide that acts by decreasing hepatic gluconeogenesis, increasing glucose uptake in peripheral tissues, and decreasing glucose absorption in the gut. Some patients find the side effects intolerable (nausea, diarrhea, flatulence). The extended release formulation of metformin, however, is often more tolerable to patients. The starting dose is 500 mg, which can be up-titrated as needed in 500-mg increments every 3–7 days (up to a maximum dose of 2,500 mg/day) as needed and as tolerated by the patient. In comparison to insulin, metformin is associated with less gestational weight gain and lower rates of both gestational hypertension and neonatal hypoglycemia (Balsells et al. 2015). Up to one-half of women treated with metformin, however, will ultimately need insulin to achieve glycemic control during pregnancy (Rowan et al. 2008).

Metformin crosses the placenta, and the long-term metabolic consequences to the offspring are unknown. A 2-year follow-up study of 211 children born to mothers who were randomly assigned treatment with insulin or metformin found no significant differences in neurodevelopmental outcomes at 2 years of age (Battin et al. 2013). As part of the same study, children had similar overall body fat composition. Those whose mothers took metformin, however, had more subcutaneous than intra-abdominal fat (Rowan et al. 2011).

Metformin should be discontinued upon achieving pregnancy in women whose only indication for taking it was ovulation induction or polycystic ovarian syndrome because RCTs have not demonstrated a benefit in reducing the incidence of spontaneous abortion or GDM and the long-term consequences of metformin are unknown in the offspring (Palomba et al. 2005, Legro et al. 2007, Vanky et al. 2010).

GLYBURIDE

Glyburide is a second-generation sulfonylurea that acts by increasing pancreatic insulin secretion as well as insulin sensitivity in peripheral tissues. The total daily dosage of glyburide is 2.5–20 mg, most commonly prescribed in two daily doses. From 4% to 16% of women on glyburide will require the addition of insulin to achieve glycemic control (Langer et al. 2000, Moore et al. 2010). Early studies of glyburide did not detect the drug in the cord serum of infants whose mothers were treated with the medication, contributing to an exponential increase in the number of women prescribed the drug after 2000 (Langer et al. 2000); however, more recent data show that glyburide does cross the placenta (Hebert et al. 2009).

Glyburide generally performs poorly when compared to both insulin and metformin with higher rates of neonatal hypoglycemia and macrosomia (Hod et al. 2015, Song et al. 2017), despite similar rates of adequate glycemic control (Langer et al. 2000). As a result, it is falling out of favor as a first-line agent for the treatment of diabetes in pregnancy. Similar to metformin, no long-term follow-up data are available in children exposed to glyburide in utero.

REFERENCES

American College of Obstetricians and Gynecologists. Practice bulletin no. 60: Clinical management guidelines for obstetrician-gynecologists. Pregestational diabetes mellitus. *Obstet Gynecol* 2005;105(3):675–685

American College of Obstetricians and Gynecologists. Practice bulletin no. 137: Gestational diabetes mellitus. *Obstet Gynecol* 2013;122(2 Pt 1):406–416

American College of Obstetricians and Gynecologists. Practice bulletin no. 190: Gestational diabetes mellitus. *Obstet Gynecol* 2018;131(2):e49–e64

American Diabetes Association. Management of diabetes in pregnancy: standards of medical care in diabetes, 2018. *Diabetes Care* 2018;41(Suppl. 1):S137–S143

Balsells M, García-Patterson A, Solà I, Roqué M, Gich I, Corcoy R. Glibenclamide, metformin, and insulin for the treatment of gestational diabetes: a systematic review and meta-analysis. *BMJ (Online)* 2015;350:h102

Battin MR, Wouldes T, Buksh M, Rowan J. Neurodevelopmental outcome at 24 months in children following a randomized trial of metformin versus insulin treatment for gestational diabetes (miG trial). *J Paediatr Child Health* 2013;49(Suppl. 2):21

Blum AK. Insulin use in pregnancy: an update. *Diabetes Spectrum* 2016;29(2): 92–97

Bonora BM, Avogaro A, Fadini GP. Exposure to insulin degludec during pregnancy: report of a small series and review of the literature. *J Endocrinol Invest* 2019;42(3):345–349. doi:10.1007/s40618-018-0926-9

Crowther CA, Hiller JE, Moss JR, McPhee AJ, Jeffries WS, Robinson JS. Effect of treatment of gestational diabetes mellitus on pregnancy outcomes. *N Engl J Med* 2005;352(24):2477–2486

Evers IM, ter Braak EW, de Valk HW, van Der Schoot B, Janssen N, Visser GH. Risk indicators predictive for severe hypoglycemia during the first trimester of type 1 diabetic pregnancy. *Diabetes Care* 2002;25(3):554–559

Feig DS, Donovan LE, Corcoy R, et al. Continuous glucose monitoring in pregnant women with type 1 diabetes (CONCEPTT): a multicentre international randomised controlled trial. *Lancet* 2017;390(10110):2347–2359

Freinkel N. Banting Lecture 1980. Of pregnancy and progeny. *Diabetes* 1980;29(12):1023–1035

Garcia-Patterson A, Gich I, Amini SB, Catalano PM, de Leiva A, Corcoy R. Insulin requirements throughout pregnancy in women with type 1 diabetes mellitus: three changes of direction. *Diabetologia* 2010;53(3):446–451

Hartling L, Dryden DM, Guthrie A, Muise M, Vandermeer B, Donovan L. Benefits and harms of treating gestational diabetes mellitus: a systematic review and meta-analysis for the U.S. preventive services task force and the National Institutes of Health Office of Medical Applications of Research. *Annals Intern Med* 2013;159(2):123–129

Hebert MF, Ma X, Naraharisetti SB, et al. Are we optimizing gestational diabetes treatment with glyburide the pharmacologic basis for better clinical practice? *Clin Pharmacol Therap* 2009;85(6):607–614

Herrera KM, Rosenn BM, Foroutan J, et al. Randomized controlled trial of insulin detemir versus NPH for the treatment of pregnant women with diabetes. *Am J Obstet Gynecol* 2015;213(3):426.e421–427

Hirsch IB. Insulin analogues. *N Engl J Med* 2005;352(2):174–183

Hod M, Kapur A, Sacks DA, et al. The International Federation of Gynecology and Obstetrics (FIGO) Initiative on gestational diabetes mellitus: a pragmatic guide for diagnosis, management, and care. *Intl J Gyn Obstet* 2015;131(S3): S173–S211

Hod M, Mathiesen ER, Jovanovič L, et al. A randomized trial comparing perinatal outcomes using insulin detemir or neutral protamine Hagedorn in type 1 diabetes. *J Mater Fetal Nenat Med* 2014;27(1):7–13

ıvanovic L. Glucose and insulin requirements during labor and delivery: the case for normoglycemia in pregnancies complicated by diabetes. *Endocrine Practice* 2004;10(Suppl. 2):40–45

Langer O, Conway DL, Berkus MD, Xenakis EM-J, Gonzales O. A comparison of glyburide and insulin in women with gestational diabetes mellitus. *N Engl J Med* 2000;343(16):1134–1138

Legro RS, Barnhart HX, Schlaff WD, et al. Clomiphene, metformin, or both for infertility in the polycystic ovary syndrome. *N Engl J Med* 2007;356(6):551–566

Mathiesen ER, Hod M, Ivanisevic M, et al. Maternal efficacy and safety outcomes in a randomized, controlled trial comparing insulin detemir with NPH insulin in 310 pregnant women with type 1 diabetes. *Diabetes Care* 2012;35(10):2012–2017

Moore LE, Clokey D, Rappaport VJ, Curet LB. Metformin compared with glyburide in gestational diabetes: a randomized controlled trial. *Obstet Gynecol* 2010;115(1):55–59

Mukhopadhyay A, Farrell T, Fraser RB, Ola B. Continuous subcutaneous insulin infusion vs intensive conventional insulin therapy in pregnant diabetic women: a systematic review and metaanalysis of randomized, controlled trials. *Am J Obstet Gynecol* 2007;197(5):447–456

National Institute for Health and Care Excellence (NICE). *Diabetes in Pregnancy: Management of Diabetes and Its Complications from Preconception to the Postnatal Period.* National Institute for Health and Clinical Excellence (NICE) National Collaborating Centre for Women's and Children's Health, 2008

National Institute for Health and Care Excellence (NICE). *Diabetes in Pregnancy: Management of Diabetes and Its Complications from Preconception to the Postnatal Period.* National Institute for Health and Clinical Excellence (NICE) National Collaborating Centre for Women's and Children's Health, 2015

O'Neill SM, Kenny LC, Khashan AS, West HM, Smyth RMD, Kearney PM. Different insulin types and regimens for pregnant women with preexisting diabetes. *Cochrane Database System Rev* 2017;2:CD011880

Palomba S, Orio Jr F, Falbo A, et al. Prospective parallel randomized, double-blind, double-dummy controlled clinical trial comparing clomiphene citrate and metformin as the first-line treatment for ovulation induction in nonobese anovulatory women with polycystic ovary syndrome. *J Clin Endrocrinol Metab* 2005;90(7):4068–4074

Ranasinghe PD, Maruthur NM, Nicholson WK, et al. Comparative effectiveness of continuous subcutaneous insulin infusion using insulin analogs and multiple daily injections in pregnant women with diabetes mellitus: a systematic review and meta-analysis. *J Women's Health* 2015;24(3):237–249

Rowan JA, Hague WM, Gao W, Battin MR, Moore MP. Metformin versus insulin for the treatment of gestational diabetes. *N Engl J Med* 2008;358(19):2003–2015

Rowan JA, Rush EC, Obolonkin V, Battin M, Wouldes T, Hague WM. Metformin in gestational diabetes: the offspring follow-up (MiG TOFU): body composition at 2 years of age. *Diabetes Care* 2011;34(10):2279–2284

Shields L, Tsay GS (Eds.). Chapter 3: Medical Management and Education for Preexisting Diabetes During Pregnancy. In *California Diabetes and Pregnancy Program Sweet Success Guidelines for Care*. California Department of Public Health; Maternal Child and Adolescent Health Division, 2015, p. 5

Society for Maternal Fetal Medicine Statement. Pharmacological treatment of gestational diabetes. *Am J Obstet Gyn* 2018;218(5):B2–B4

Song R, Chen L, Chen Y, et al. Comparison of glyburide and insulin in the management of gestational diabetes: a meta-analysis. *PLoS One* 2017; 12(8):e0182488

Trujillo AL. Insulin analogs and pregnancy. *Diabetes Spectrum* 2007;20(2):94–101

Vanky E, Stridsklev S, Heimstad R, et al. Metformin versus placebo from first trimester to delivery in polycystic ovary syndrome: a randomized, controlled multicenter study. *J Clin Endocrinol Metab* 2010;95(12):E448–E455

Wang H, Wender-Ozegowska E, Garne E, et al. Insulin analogues use in pregnancy among women with pregestational diabetes mellitus and risk of congenital anomaly: a retrospective population-based cohort study. *BMJ Open* 2018;8(2):e014972. doi:10.1136/ bmjopen-2016-014972

Risk Assessment, Fetal Surveillance, and Delivery in Pregnancies Complicated by Diabetes

Highlights

Screening, Diagnostic Testing, and Fetal Surveillance

Genetic Screening

Ultrasound

Antenatal Testing

Timing and Mode of Delivery

Selected Readings

References

Highlights
Risk Assessment, Fetal Surveillance, and Delivery in Pregnancies Complicated by Diabetes

■ Screening with maternal serum α-fetoprotein, multiple-marker screening, or cell-free DNA testing can identify some fetal aneuploidies and open fetal defects.

■ Diagnostic genetic testing with modalities, such as amniocentesis and chorionic villus sampling, should be offered to all patients, particularly those with abnormal screening tests.

■ Diagnostic genetic testing with amniocentesis and chorionic villus sampling also can be used to detect many inherited disorders; genetic counseling allows for the determination of which disorders these tests should target.

■ Ultrasound is useful in determining gestational age, evaluating fetal anatomy, assessing fetal growth and weight, and determining fetal well-being during an antepartum biophysical profile.

■ Antepartum fetal status can be determined through the evaluation of the fetal heart rate pattern. Antenatal testing has reduced the necessity for preterm delivery of infants of mothers with diabetes.

■ Patients with well-controlled diabetes do not necessarily require preterm delivery or even delivery before 39 weeks, assuming no other complications and normal antenatal testing.

■ Gestational diabetes mellitus (GDM) is not a contraindication to vaginal delivery. In women with both preexisting diabetes and GDM, mode of delivery should be based on the clinical scenario and cesarean delivery reserved for obstetric indications or sonographic estimated fetal weight >4,500 g.

Risk Assessment, Fetal Surveillance, and Delivery in Pregnancies Complicated by Diabetes

Screening, diagnostic testing, and fetal surveillance include various modalities of testing performed at various time points during pregnancy so that fetal development may be assessed (Table 5.1). It is important that both caregivers and patients understand that tests that can and will ensure the birth of a perfectly "healthy" baby do not exist; furthermore, one can only look for known problems with specific tests. Therefore, assurances that "everything will be fine" should be avoided no matter how many normal test results are reported.

GENETIC SCREENING

The American College of Obstetricians and Gynecologists (ACOG) recommends that all women be offered screening or diagnostic testing for aneuploidy and genetic disorders. Although maternal diabetes does not increase the risk for genetically inherited diseases, like all prenatal patients, individuals with diabetes should be questioned about family history, including ethnic background, with an eye toward the identification of genetic risk factors. For example, patients of Ashkenazi Jewish or French Canadian descent are at increased risk of being carriers for Tay-Sachs disease, a uniformly fatal autosomal recessive disorder. Additionally, maternal age is associated with an increased risk for chromosomal abnormalities. It is important to note that diabetes does not change the relationship between maternal age and the risk of aneuploidy; however, mothers at the age of 35 years have an ~1 in 180 chance of delivering a baby with a chromosomal abnormality and about half of these babies will be born with Down's syndrome. Thus, any patients for whom age or family history suggests increased risk of genetic disorders should receive thorough genetic counseling. Several testing and diagnostic options are available to patients (ACOG 2016a, 2016b).

Alpha-fetoprotein (αFP), a fetal product that appears in both amniotic fluid and maternal circulation, often is present in increased concentration when an open fetal defect occurs (i.e., anencephaly, neural tube defect, spinal defect, or ventral wall defect, such as omphalocele or gastroschisis). Because maternal type 1 diabetes (T1D) is associated with an increased risk for congenital malformations, maternal serum αFP (MSαFP) screening is generally offered to these patients. Maternal concentrations of αFP may be low in some cases of chromosomal aneuploidy (i.e., trisomy 21). αFP screening is most accurate

Table 5.1—Screening, Diagnostic Testing, and Fetal Surveillance

Test	Purpose	Optimal Gestational Age	Comments
Ultrasound	Establish gestational age	After 6 weeks	Reliability: 6–8 weeks 6 days: ±5 days 9–15 weeks 6 days: ±7 days 16–21 weeks 6 days: ±10 days 22–27 weeks 6 days: ±14 days >28 weeks: ±21 days
	Screen for structural anomalies	Variable	Detects many anomalies but cannot guarantee normalcy
	Detect macrosomia and hydramnios	26 weeks to term	Identification of fetal effects of gestational diabetes mellitus
α-fetoprotein (αFP)	Detect risk of open fetal defect	15–20 weeks	If elevated, possible open fetal defect (e.g., anencephaly, spina bifida)
Integrated screen, multiple markers, with or without nuchal translucency	Detect risk of certain aneuploidies	Part 1: 10 weeks 3 days to 13 weeks; part 2: 15–22 weeks 6 days	Detects risk of trisomy 21, 18, 13, and open fetal defects
Cell-free fetal DNA testing of maternal blood	Test for trisomy 13, 18, 21, and monosomy X	>9 weeks	Indeterminate or uninterpretable results need further evaluation
Genetic testing on maternal or paternal blood sample	Detect carrier state for heritable diseases	Any	Looks for a specific disease; currently available for Tay-Sachs, cystic fibrosis, sickle cell disease, thalassemia, and many others
Genetic amniocentesis	Test for chromosome abnormalities	>15 weeks	Small risk of complications; diabetes does not increase the risk of chromosomal abnormalities
Chorionic villus sampling	Test for chromosome abnormalities	>9 weeks	Increased miscarriage rate
Fetal activity	Screen for fetal well-being	28–40 weeks	Simple, inexpensive
Nonstress test	Screen for fetal well-being	26–40 weeks	Risk of false positives in a sleeping, immature, or inactive fetus

Table 5.1 (continued)

Test	Purpose	Optimal Gestational Age	Comments
Biophysical profile	Evaluate chronic and acute fetal problems using ultrasound	26–40 weeks	Potentially the most reliable
Amniocentesis	Test for fetal lung maturity	Preterm	Not often needed
Doppler velocimetry	Test for fetal umbilical blood flow in fetal growth restriction (FGR)	Third trimester	Assessment of the risk of fetal demise in FGR, not recommended in appropriately grown fetuses

at ~15–20 weeks of gestation, and thus that is the ideal time for maternal serum screening. To standardize results, the MSαFP level is expressed by the laboratory in multiples of the median (MOM). Various centers recommend further testing at levels ≥2.0 or >2.5 MOM. At a given gestational age, women with T1D have been reported to manifest lower MSαFP when compared with women who do not have diabetes. Some studies have linked this lowering of MSαFP to poor metabolic control as manifested by elevated hemoglobin A_{1c} (A1C) levels. Depending on the circumstances and patient preference, an elevated MSαFP may prompt either an amniocentesis (to measure amniotic fluid αFP) or an extended fetal anatomic survey (ACOG 2016a, 2016b, 2018b).

In addition to αFP, most centers offer multiple-marker screening, in which measurements of the levels of substances other than αFP, such as human chorionic gonadotropin (hCG) and estriol, are used to predict the risk for chromosomal aneuploidies. Because maternal diabetes does not appear to increase the risk for such aneuploidies in the fetus, these multiple-marker tests should be considered equally appropriate for women with diabetes as for the general population. A further refinement in the area of genetic screening combines first-trimester screening (nuchal translucency measurement with or without serum markers, including PAPP-A, and β-hCG) with multiple-marker screening in the second trimester (αFP, unconjugated estriol, inhibin-A, and β-hCG). When results of first-trimester screening are combined with those of second-trimester screening to provide a single risk estimate, the test is called an "integrated screen." When first-trimester screening results are conveyed so that high-risk results can lead to further diagnostic testing while lower-risk results can be refined by second-trimester screening, the test is called a "sequential screen." Further details are beyond the scope of this chapter, but readers are referred to ACOG Practice Bulletins on the topic, numbers 162 and 163 (ACOG 2016a, 2016b).

Cell-free fetal DNA screening is a relatively new technology used to assess a pregnancy for the risk of aneuploidy. Fetal DNA circulates in the maternal bloodstream and can be detected as early as 9 weeks of gestation. A number of techniques have been developed that are able to use this circulating cell-free DNA to screen for fetal aneuploidy. These screens have high sensitivity and specificity for trisomy 18 and trisomy 21; they also can be used to assess the risk of trisomy 13, determine fetal sex, determine fetal Rh status, and detect some paternally derived autosomal dominant genetic conditions. Because the amount of fetal DNA in the bloodstream increases throughout pregnancy, the test can be run as early as 9 weeks and at any time up until delivery. Originally designed for use in a high-risk population, cell-free DNA screening can be offered to all patients regardless of baseline risk. It is important, however, that women who have results that are "not reported," "indeterminate," "uninterpretable," or "no call" receive further genetic counseling and are offered diagnostic testing because an "indeterminate" result represents an increased risk of aneuploidy (ACOG 2016b).

To this point, the aforementioned options are considered screening tests. When a screening test is positive, patients first must be counseled on the ramifications and limitations of the positive findings and then confirmatory diagnostic testing should be offered. There are two well-studied diagnostic testing strategies: chorionic villus sampling (CVS) and amniocentesis.

CVS involves taking a "biopsy" of the placenta; this is taken either through a catheter inserted into the uterus transvaginally or with a needle inserted transabdominally. CVS is available only in specialized centers. Its advantages include that it can be accomplished earlier in pregnancy than amniocentesis, as early as 9 weeks, and that the results can be available in just a few days. For some couples, this decreases decision-making pressure, because first-trimester pregnancy terminations are safer and less traumatic to the mother. The primary disadvantage of CVS is that there is an increased pregnancy loss rate reported compared with amniocentesis, and a few case series have reported an excess of limb defects in the offspring born to mothers who had CVS testing, particularly with very early CVS and with inexperienced operators. Thus, couples interested in CVS should be referred to experienced centers and should undergo extensive counseling before the procedure (ACOG 2016a).

Genetic amniocentesis, the most common method of genetic diagnostic testing, is a procedure during which, under ultrasound guidance, a needle is inserted transabdominally into the amniotic sac to obtain amniotic fluid. Fetal cells separated from the amniotic fluid are grown in tissue culture for karyotyping (chromosome analysis) or other types of testing. Amniocentesis is generally performed at 14–20 weeks of gestation, and the results of metaphase analysis of cultured cells may take anywhere from 1–2 weeks to return, depending on the tests desired and the laboratory facilities. Fluorescence in situ hybridization (FISH) analysis can provide more rapid results when specific chromosome number defects, such as those involving chromosome 21, 13, 18, or the sex chromosomes, are sought. False-negative and false-positive results may occur with FISH testing, however, so these results should be confirmed by karyotyping or the presence of other evidence, such as ultrasound markers for the particular defect, or positive screening tests. Several different enzymatic defects also can be determined from fetal cells in amniotic fluid, but each requires the services of a specialized laboratory. Thus, it is necessary to know whether a particular couple is at risk for a particular genetic disease; there is no screening test on amniotic fluid that can detect all of the possible genetic diseases (ACOG 2016a). There is a small but definite risk of an adverse event, such as premature labor, rupture of the membranes, or fetal injury associated with amniocentesis, with a perinatal loss rate estimated at between

1 in 300 and 1 in 500. Thus, patients should be informed of these risks before the procedure. Further information on invasive prenatal testing may be found in an ACOG Practice Bulletin (ACOG 2016a).

Amniocentesis also can be used later in pregnancy to assess fetal lung maturity. Several early studies suggested that respiratory distress syndrome (RDS), which histologically manifests as hyaline membrane disease, occurs with increased frequency and at later gestational ages in infants of mothers with diabetes. Tissue culture experiments have linked this problem to fetal hyperinsulinemia, brought about by suboptimal maternal metabolic control. Conversely, however, subsequent reports suggest that the risk for RDS is closer to background rates when maternal diabetes is well controlled (Kjos et al. 1990). The use of amniotic fluid biochemical analysis can identify fetuses at greatest risk for RDS if delivered as well as fetuses highly unlikely to develop this complication. At one time, amniocentesis was quite useful in evaluating lung maturity in the fetus of a mother with diabetes. A workshop in 2011, sponsored by the National Institute of Child Health and Human Development and the Society for Maternal–Fetal Medicine, however, recommended that amniocentesis rarely be used to determine the timing of delivery in pregnancies complicated by maternal diabetes (Spong et al. 2011). The rationale was that if clinical concern for fetal well-being is heightened enough to recommend delivery because of poor glucose control, vascular, or other complications, fetal lung maturation status likely should not dissuade providers from delivery as RDS can be treated postnatally with good long-term survival (Spong et al. 2011).

ULTRASOUND

Ultrasound has widespread application in obstetrics, particularly in the evaluation and management of the high-risk pregnancy. Because accurate dating of pregnancy is critical to improve outcomes as well as to plan for various evaluations and interventions during pregnancy, the earliest application of ultrasound in pregnancy is its use in establishing the estimated date of delivery (EDD; the due date).

Around 6 weeks of menstrual age (time elapsed since the first day of the last menstrual period), using standard transabdominal ultrasound equipment, the presence or absence of a gestational sac and fetal pole can be demonstrated. Between 6 weeks and 13 weeks 6 days of gestation, the crown-rump length of the fetus can be measured, with an accuracy of ±5–7 days for one measurement. If multiple measurements are taken, the accuracy is increased (ACOG 2017).

After 14 weeks of gestation, dating is usually accomplished using a variety of ultrasound measurements, including the biparietal diameter and circumference of the fetal head, the abdominal circumference, and the fetal femur length. The accuracy of these measurements is ±7 days between 14 weeks and 16 weeks 6 days, ±10 days between 17 weeks and 21 weeks 6 days, and ±14 days between 22 weeks and 27 weeks 6 days. If ultrasound-estimated gestational age is within such confidence intervals based on last menstrual period, it is customary not to change the EDD, assuming that the patient is relatively certain about her last menstrual period and that her menses follow a fairly consistent pattern and length. After 28 weeks of gestation, ultrasound estimates of gestational age diminish in reliability because of the large week-to-week overlap in the measurements taken (American Academy of Pediatrics 2017; ACOG 2016c, 2017).

Once gestational age has been established, ultrasound can be used to screen for fetal aneuploidy. The nuchal translucency is the fluid-filled space on the back of the fetal neck. Between 10 weeks and 13 weeks 6 days of gestation ultrasound is used to measure this space. An enlarged nuchal translucency (≥3.0 mm) is associated with fetal malformations and aneuploidy (ACOG 2016b).

Ultrasound can also be used to evaluate fetal anatomy. The use of fetal ultrasound for detection of congenital anomalies is suggested for women with preexisting diabetes as well as for women with GDM who are suspected of having preexisting diabetes (A1C values ≥6.5%, fasting plasma glucose levels ≥126 mg/dL [≥7.0 mmol/L], or random glucose ≥200 mg/dL [11.1 mmol/L] at first visit). The presence of maternal diabetes carries with it a significant increase in the likelihood of major congenital malformations; indeed, these occur in 6–12% of infants born to mothers with preexisting diabetes. Hyperglycemia during organogenesis carries the highest risk. Although not all malformations can be diagnosed with ultrasound, many can be found with a thorough sonographic fetal evaluation. Therefore, detailed ultrasound studies (also known as level II ultrasound or targeted ultrasound) should be carried out in pregnancies complicated by diabetes, especially in cases in which other risk factors are known to be present. Such risk factors include an elevated A1C at the time of first prenatal visit, high or low serum or amniotic fluid αFP, or a personal or family history of delivering an infant with anomalies. Unfortunately, a negative result in no way guarantees fetal normalcy, and patients should be informed of the limitations of ultrasound before scanning commences (ACOG 2016c).

In addition to verifying gestational age and identifying major anatomic abnormalities in the fetus, ultrasound is a useful tool for the assessment of fetal growth and the estimation of fetal weight. Because the fetus of a mother with diabetes may be macrosomic (large for gestational age) or alternatively may be growth restricted (small for gestational age), particularly in the presence of maternal vascular disease or hypertension, it is useful to perform periodic measurements of fetal growth during the third trimester. Excessive amounts of amniotic fluid (polyhydramnios) also may complicate diabetic pregnancy and usually can be detected with ultrasound (Coomarasamy et al. 2005, Langer 2005, Chauhan et al. 2006, Nahum and Stanislaw 2006, Farrell et al. 2007, ACOG 2018b).

ANTENATAL TESTING

Antenatal fetal testing is routinely used to assess the risk of adverse outcomes and fetal demise in pregnancies complicated by maternal conditions, such as hypertension or diabetes. In pregnancies complicated by maternal diabetes, decisions regarding the commencement, type, and frequency of surveillance for fetal well-being should be influenced by the severity of maternal hyperglycemia and the presence of other adverse clinical factors, such as past poor obstetric history or coincident hypertensive disorders. Several antenatal fetal surveillance techniques exist, and they range from maternal perception of fetal movement (FM) to contraction stress test and umbilical artery Doppler velocimetry (ACOG 2014).

The nonstress test (NST) is an assessment of fetal well-being based on observations from prior research that the healthy fetus usually demonstrates a transient increase in its heart rate after any vigorous FM. The presence of two to three such accelerations with an increase of at least 15 beats/min, lasting at least 15 s, during a 20-min period is associated with a high likelihood of fetal well-being and is called a reactive NST (Figure 5.1). Because the NST requires only an electronic fetal monitor, it is easy to perform and often is used as a primary test of fetal well-being. A reactive NST is a strong indicator of fetal well-being, but a nonreactive NST may be seen in fetal sleep states, fetal immaturity, and other situations that are not necessarily adverse. Thus, a nonreactive NST is usually followed up by another fetoplacental function test, such as a biophysical profile (ACOG 2014).

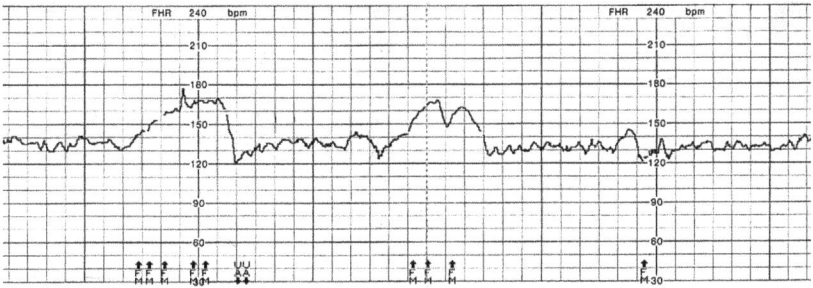

Figure 5.1—Fetal monitor strip from NST. Note the rise in fetal heart rate (FHR) with each fetal movement (FM).

The biophysical profile is thought to combine the evaluation of chronic and acute fetal problems. In this test, the NST is combined with an ultrasound evaluation of FM, fetal tone (flexion of the extremities), amniotic fluid volume, and fetal breathing. Each category is assigned a score of 0 (bad) or 2 (good) points. A score of 8–10 is normal; a score of 6 is equivocal and suggests possible fetal jeopardy or asphyxia; and a score of 0–4 is abnormal and very strongly indicative of fetal compromise (ACOG 2014). The presence of oligohydramnios (amniotic fluid index [AFI] ≤5 cm or deepest vertical pocket ≤2 cm) is highly suggestive of chronic problems (or ruptured membranes) and requires further evaluation or delivery, depending on the gestational age and clinical circumstances. The modified biophysical profile includes an NST plus the measurement of the AFI. If both are normal, no further evaluation is needed at that time. If either or both are abnormal, further evaluation is recommended (ACOG 2014).

Each time the uterus contracts during normal labor, the delivery of nutrients and oxygen to the fetus is diminished. Ordinarily, the fetus possesses sufficient redundancy in its reserves of these substances such that the contraction has no ill effect. A fetus functioning "on the edge," however, with depleted placental reserves, may respond to each uterine contraction with a characteristic slowing of its heart rate, technically known as a "late deceleration" when viewed on an electronic printout monitoring fetal heart rate (FHR) (Figure 5.2). Such late decelerations, if repetitive, are considered to be nonreassuring, possibly reflecting fetal compromise during labor. Similar changes may be seen on FHR tracings of pregnant women who are not yet in spontaneous labor but who have had contractions artificially induced with an intravenous infusion of oxytocin. The oxytocin challenge test consists of the induction of at least three uterine contractions during a 10-min period. If all three contractions are followed by late decelerations of the FHR, the test is considered positive and indicative of a high likelihood of fetal compromise (ACOG 2014).

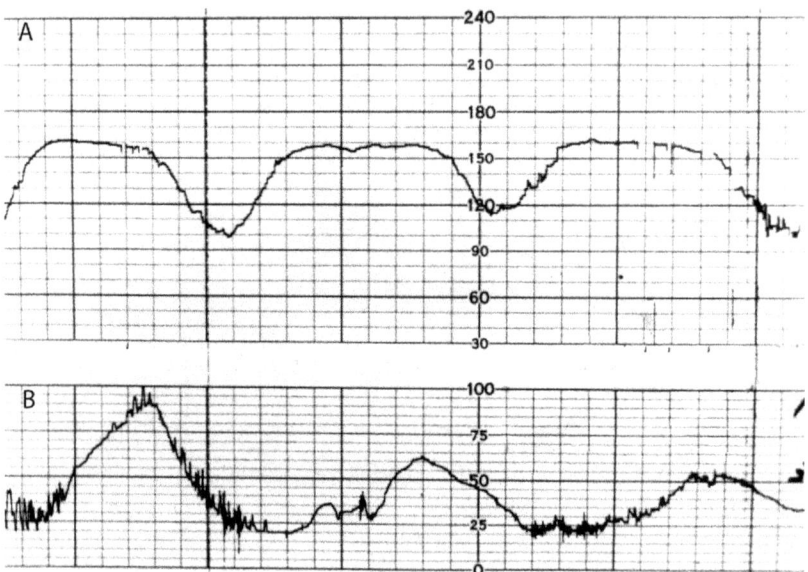

Figure 5.2—Late decelerations. A: Fetal heart rate; **B:** uterine contractions. Note the fetal heart rate dip to 100 beats/min after contraction.

Doppler ultrasound is used in pregnancies complicated by fetal growth restriction (FGR). It is a noninvasive test that allows for evaluation of vascular resistance in the placenta. It has been established that flow velocity waveforms in the umbilical artery of a growth-restricted fetus are different than those of a normally grown fetus. In pregnancies complicated by FGR, umbilical artery Doppler studies provide an additional assessment of fetal well-being. Umbilical artery diastolic flow in a normal pregnancy is high velocity flow, whereas in a fetus with FGR, umbilical artery diastolic flow is decreased. Umbilical artery diastolic flow in a fetus with FGR that is absent or reversed represents an increased risk of perinatal mortality. At this time, no data have demonstrated that Doppler ultrasound is informative when used to evaluate a normally grown fetus; thus, it is reserved for pregnancies complicated by FGR. Pregnancies complicated by diabetes, particularly those with evidence of vascular disease, are at risk for both macrosomia and FGR and, hence, monthly growth ultrasounds are routinely performed. Weekly Doppler ultrasounds, however, are reserved for cases of FGR (ACOG 2014).

Different perinatal centers use different combinations of these antenatal tests when evaluating a pregnant woman with diabetes. There is no single approach on which there is universal agreement, and data are not available to demonstrate which method is superior. Certain principles, however, are generally accepted. Most centers would not start any type of antenatal testing until a gestational age is reached at which there is a possibility of fetal survival if delivery is accomplished (no testing <23 weeks of gestation). Because all of these methods of antenatal fetal surveillance can yield false-positive results, they should not be performed if a particular patient has little risk of fetal problems; in such patients, the predictive accuracy of a positive test is poor. Thus, a particular center might defer antenatal testing until 35 weeks in a patient with well-controlled diabetes who has no vascular complications, but might start at 28 weeks or even earlier in a patient with poorly controlled diabetes who also has nephropathy, hypertension, and a growth-restricted fetus. The interval of testing may vary from once per week to daily depending on the circumstances of a particular patient. Whatever approach is taken, tests should be performed in a center in which there is adequate day-to-day experience in the performance and interpretation of the selected modalities (ACOG 2014).

As a general rule, among women with preexisting diabetes, it is appropriate to initiate antenatal fetal testing twice per week at 32 weeks of gestation. Clinical guidelines should never be used as a substitute for clinical judgment—for example, as mentioned earlier, sooner testing may be necessary at 28 weeks or even earlier in a poorly controlled patient with diabetes who also has other high-risk conditions (ACOG 2014, 2018b).

With regard to women with GDM, ACOG has suggested that a reasonable approach would be to manage patients with GDM who require insulin, patients whose GDM is not well controlled, or patients who have other risk factors, such as a poor obstetric history or hypertension, in the same way as individuals with preexisting diabetes (ACOG 2018a). Data are insufficient to determine whether surveillance beyond self-monitoring of FM is indicated in women with GDM who meet the targets of glycemic control with diet alone and in whom fetal growth is appropriate for gestational age (ACOG 2018a).

TIMING AND MODE OF DELIVERY

At one time, it was common to deliver infants born to mothers with diabetes at some arbitrary number of weeks before term to lessen the likelihood of unexplained fetal demise in utero. Because of the need for early delivery when the uterine cervix was not yet "ripe" to facilitate induction of labor and because fetal macrosomia complicated a significant proportion of these pregnancies, cesarean delivery was the routine route of birth. The advent of antenatal testing, as described in this chapter, allows for the identification of particular pregnancies at high risk for impending intrauterine fetal demise, so that the less threatened fetuses may be allowed to continue closer to term. Most important, modern approaches to metabolic normalization of the pregnant woman with diabetes have prevented fetal deterioration, and as a result, early delivery is less likely to be necessary. Because pregnancies allowed to progress closer to term are more likely to result in vaginal delivery and because improved metabolic control has lowered, but not eliminated, the likelihood of fetal macrosomia, women with diabetes often can safely deliver vaginally (Spong et al. 2011; ACOG 2018a, 2018b).

Timing of delivery will depend on clinical scenario (Table 5.2); however, in women with well-controlled diabetes, no evidence of vascular complications, and normal antenatal testing, delivery is generally recommended between 39 and

40 weeks of gestation (Spong et al. 2011, ACOG 2018b). Among women with evidence of vascular complications, however, even if well controlled, delivery may be considered between 37 weeks and 39 weeks 6 days of gestation (Spong et al. 2011). In patients with poor glucose control, multiple comorbidities, or prior poor obstetric outcomes, such as stillbirth, early delivery may be indicated to balance the risk of fetal demise with that of preterm birth; these cases must be individualized depending on the clinical scenario. As noted, when delivery before 39 weeks is determined to be the safest course, amniocentesis is not recommended (Spong et al. 2011, ACOG 2018b).

With regard to women with GDM, recommendations regarding timing of delivery are slightly different. A retrospective study of all births to women with GDM in California delivering from 1997 through 2006 compared the infant mortality risk associated with delivery at a given gestational age to the risks of stillbirth plus infant mortality associated with waiting 1 more week to deliver (Rosenstein et al. 2012). The risk of expectant management was lower than that of delivery at 36 weeks, although the difference was not statistically significant. At 37 and 38 weeks, the risks were similar. At 39 and 40 weeks, the risks of expectant management of GDM for 1 more week were significantly higher than for delivery. For example, the mortality risk of delivery at 39 weeks was 8.7/10,000 versus 17.1/10,000 if the pregnancy was managed expectantly for 1 more week. The authors calculated that 1,311 patients with GDM would need to be delivered at 39 weeks to prevent one excess stillbirth (Rosenstein et al. 2012, ACOG 2018a). Thus, a policy of delivery between 39 and 40 weeks appears appropriate for patients with well-controlled GDM. ACOG recommends that among women with GDM well controlled by diet, no other high-risk issues, and normal antepartum testing, expectant management up until 40 weeks 6 days of gestation is reasonable. Among women with medication-controlled GDM, without other issues and normal testing, delivery is recommended between 39 weeks and 39 weeks 6 days of gestation (ACOG 2018a). If, however, women have poorly controlled GDM, late preterm (34–36 weeks +6/7 days) or early term (37–38 weeks +6/7 days) delivery may be indicated depending on the individual clinical scenario (Spong et al. 2011, ACOG 2018a).

Table 5.2—Timing of Delivery in Women with Diabetes in Pregnancy

Type of Diabetes	Glucose Control	Complications	Delivery Timing
Preexisting diabetes	Well controlled	None	39 weeks
	Well controlled	Significant	37–39 weeks
	Suboptimal	None	37–39 weeks
	Suboptimal	Significant	34–39 weeks
Gestational diabetes mellitus	Well controlled by diet	None	39–40 weeks
	Well controlled by medication	None	39 weeks
	Suboptimal	None	37–39 weeks
	Suboptimal	Significant	34–39 weeks

Source: Adapted from ACOG (2019).

In women with both preexisting diabetes and GDM, the mode of delivery should be based on the clinical scenario. Diabetes is not a contraindication to vaginal delivery. As a general rule, cesarean delivery should be reserved for obstetric indications, such as malpresentation, history of shoulder dystocia, labor dystocia, and history of multiple prior cesarean deliveries (>2). In the case of a sonographic estimated fetal weight of >4,500 g, to prevent birth trauma, cesarean delivery should be considered and offered (ACOG 2018a, 2018b).

During labor, both maternal and fetal monitoring is recommended for women with pregnancies complicated by both preexisting diabetes and GDM. Because preexisting diabetes and, to a lesser extent, GDM represent a pregnancy with increased baseline risk of fetal compromise, intrapartum continuous electronic fetal monitoring should be utilized once labor has been established (ACOG 2014, 2018a, 2018b).

During labor, frequent assessment of maternal capillary glucose is recommended to prevent maternal hyperglycemia, fetal hypoxia, and neonatal hypoglycemia. Among women with T1D and type 2 diabetes (T2D), glucose levels should be checked hourly with the goal that maternal glucose be maintained somewhere between 70 and 100 mg/dL. During labor, women may not require insulin; however, if necessary, insulin and dextrose infusions may be utilized to control maternal blood glucose (Montoro 2004, ACOG 2018b). With regard to women with GDM, there is a paucity of data and guidelines guiding intrapartum glucose management. Most management regimens have been extrapolated from guidelines for women with preexisting diabetes. Although most providers agree that maternal glucose levels should be monitored intrapartum, the frequency of testing and goal glucose levels vary by provider and institution. Prospective studies are needed to determine the frequency of measurement and the optimal glucose levels that are associated with the best perinatal outcome among pregnancies complicated by GDM (ACOG 2018a, 2018b).

SELECTED READINGS

American College of Obstetricians and Gynecologists. Committee opinion no. 693: Counseling about genetic testing and communication of genetic test results. *Obstet Gynecol* 2017;129:e96–e101

REFERENCES

American Academy of Pediatrics and the American College of Obstetricians and Gynecologists. *Guidelines for Perinatal Care*. 8th ed. Washington, DC, AAP and ACOG, 2017, chapters 5–7

American College of Obstetricians and Gynecologists. Practice bulletin no. 145: Antepartum fetal surveillance. *Obstet Gynecol* 2014;124:182–192 (reaffirmed 2016)

American College of Obstetricians and Gynecologists. Practice bulletin no. 162: Prenatal diagnostic testing for genetic disorders. *Obstet Gynecol* 2016a;127:e108–e122

American College of Obstetricians and Gynecologists. Practice bulletin no. 163: Screening for fetal aneuploidy. *Obstet Gynecol* 2016b;127:e123–e137

American College of Obstetricians and Gynecologists. Practice bulletin no. 175: Ultrasound in pregnancy. *Obstet Gynecol* 2016c;128:e241–e156

American College of Obstetricians and Gynecologists. Committee opinion no. 700: Methods for estimating the due date. *Obstet Gynecol* 2017;129:e150–e154

American College of Obstetricians and Gynecologists. Practice bulletin no. 190: Gestational diabetes mellitus. *Obstet Gynecol* 2018a;131:e49–e64

American College of Obstetricians and Gynecologists. Practice bulletin no. 201: Preexisting diabetes mellitus. *Obstet Gynecol* 2018b;132:e228–e248

American College of Obstetricians and Gynecologists. Committee opinion no. 764: Medically indicated late pre-term and early-term deliveries. *Obstet Gynecol* 2019;133:e151–e155

Chauhan SP, Parker D, Shields D, Sanderson M, Cole JH, Scardo JA. Sonographic estimate of birth weight among high-risk patients: feasibility and factors influencing accuracy. *Am J Obstet Gynecol* 2006;195:601–606

Coomarasamy A, Connock M, Thornton J, Khan KS. Accuracy of ultrasound biometry in the prediction of macrosomia: a systematic quantitative review. *Br J Obstet Gynaecol* 2005;112:1461–1466

Farrell T, Owen P, Kernaghan D, Ola B, Bruce C, Fraser R. Can ultrasound fetal biometry predict fetal hyperinsulinaemia at delivery in pregnancy complicated by maternal diabetes? *Eur J Obstet Gyncol Reprod Biol* 2007;131:146–150

Kjos SL, Walther FJ, Montoro M, et al. Prevalence and etiology of respiratory distress syndrome in infants of diabetic mothers: predictive value of fetal lung maturation tests. *Am J Obstet Gynecol* 1990;163:898–903

Langer O. Ultrasound biometry evolves in the management of diabetes in pregnancy. *Ultrasound Obstet Gynecol* 2005;26:585–595

Montoro MM. Diabetic ketoacidosis in pregnancy. In *Diabetes in Women: Adolescence, Pregnancy, and Menopause*. Reece EA, Coustan DR, Gabbe SG, Eds. Philadelphia, PA, Lippincott Williams & Wilkins, 2004, p. 345–350

Nahum GG, Stanislaw H. Accurate prediction of fetal macrosomia using combination methods. *Am J Obstet Gynecol* 2006;195:879–880

Rosenstein MG, Cheng YW, Snowden JM, et al. The risk of stillbirth and infant death stratified by gestational age in women with gestational diabetes. *Am J Obstet Gynecol* 2012;206:309.e1–e7

Spong CY, Mercer BM, D'Alton M, Kilpatrick S, Blackwell S, Saade G. Timing of indicated late-preterm and early-term birth. *Obstet Gynecol* 2011;118:323–333

Common Complications of Diabetes in Pregnancy

Highlights
Common Complications of Diabetes in Pregnancy

■ Hyperemesis is common in pregnancy and can be particularly challenging in women with diabetes requiring insulin.

■ Preterm birth occurs more commonly in women with diabetes. Antenatal corticosteroids, especially before 34 weeks of gestation, are important to improve neonatal outcomes, but they can increase maternal hyperglycemia in the short term.

■ The longer a woman has had diabetes, the greater her risk of developing preeclampsia in pregnancy. The Task Force Report "Hypertension in Pregnancy," issued by the American College of Obstetricians and Gynecologists in 2013, reviewed available data and reported evidence-based recommendations for the prevention, diagnosis, and treatment of preeclampsia.

Common Complications of Diabetes in Pregnancy

The Centers for Disease Control and Prevention reported that the rate of diabetes in reproductive-age women between 18 and 44 years old increased from 2.1% in 2001 to 2.9% in 2009. By 2015, approximately 4.6 million Americans 18–44 years old had diabetes, meaning that about half of them were women of reproductive age. As a consequence of the increasing prevalence of diabetes among reproductive-age adults, preexisting diabetes is becoming a more frequent complication of pregnancy. As such, both the endocrinologist and obstetrician must be familiar with the management of preexisting diabetes during pregnancy, including common complications that may arise.

HYPEREMESIS AND GASTROPARESIS

Morning sickness—nausea or vomiting during pregnancy—is one of the most common symptoms of early pregnancy, affecting 50–80% of pregnant women (American College of Obstetricians and Gynecologists [ACOG] 2018a). It is usually a tolerable annoyance for most women, but for pregnant patients with diabetes, the management of morning sickness requires special attention.

The cause of morning sickness is not completely understood, although relaxation of the smooth muscle of the stomach probably plays a role. The rapid rise of human chorionic gonadotropin (hCG) also has been implicated, because the highest prevalence of nausea and vomiting occurs at a time in pregnancy when hCG levels are at their peak. Although in the past various theories have been put forth invoking a psychological cause of hyperemesis gravidarum, evidence for such an etiology is unconvincing (Buckwalter and Simpson 2002). Hyperemesis gravidarum is the most extreme manifestation of nausea and vomiting. It usually is diagnosed in the presence of persistent nausea and vomiting without another cause, accompanied by significant weight loss (5% of prepregnancy weight) and a measure of starvation (ketonuria). Liver function tests, thyroid function tests, and electrolytes may also be abnormal (ACOG 2018a). Hyperemesis gravidarum is associated with molar pregnancy, which often manifests with hCG levels in the hundreds of thousands. The association between female sex of the fetus and hyperemesis gravidarum is not understood but is a known fact. In a retrospective study based on case notes of 166 women hospitalized for hyperemesis (Tan et al. 2006), female fetuses were significantly associated with severe starvation ketonemia and high urea. When vomiting resulted in severe dehydration during pregnancy, 85% of the fetuses were female (Tan et al. 2006).

Hyperemesis is rarely caused by hyperthyroidism, but far more often hyperthyroidism is wrongly diagnosed in the first trimester of pregnancy. Thyroid-stimulating hormone (TSH) is normally suppressed, sometimes to the level of undetectability, in the first trimester because of its structural similarity to hCG. Thus, low TSH in the first trimester is physiologic, not pathologic. If there is high suspicion for thyroid disease, free thyroid hormone levels should be performed because TSH alone is not diagnostic.

Typically, the symptoms of hyperemesis begin before 9 weeks of gestation. The degree of nausea or vomiting a patient experiences and the sights or smells that trigger it can vary greatly from one pregnancy to another, although women who have had the problem before are more likely to experience it again. Symptoms are often more severe with multifetal gestations. A search for underlying causes should be considered when symptoms manifest after 9 weeks, or when other symptoms such as pain, tenderness, or fever are present; in women with diabetes, gastroparesis should be high on the differential diagnosis list. Hyperthyroidism, gastrointestinal disorders, and genitourinary disorders also may cause hyperemesis.

NONPHARMACOLOGIC TREATMENTS

Special attention should be paid in a woman with diabetes with hyperemesis gravidarum to ensure strict glucose control and hydration to prevent first-trimester complications associated with diabetes. The treatment of morning sickness is seldom so successful that a woman will have complete relief. Time seems to be the only real cure. Women taking multivitamins at the time of conception are less likely to experience nausea and vomiting (Czeizel et al. 1992, Emelianova et al. 1999). Dietary changes may minimize the discomfort and make the situation at least manageable (Table 6.1), although evidence is lacking for most of these interventions. In a systematic review of published studies, ginger capsules (250–1,500 mg/day) have been shown to improve nausea and vomiting (Borrelli et al. 2005).

Nausea usually is worse when the stomach is empty—hence, the early morning symptoms. For this reason, it is suggested that patients keep some starch, such as melba toast, rice cakes, saltines, or other low-fat crackers, at the bedside so they can eat if they become nauseated in the middle of the night or before getting out of bed in the morning. Eating a protein and carbohydrate snack at bedtime, such as cheese and crackers or half of a sandwich, will help prevent early morning nausea. This snack also helps prevent the development of ketonuria, which may aggravate nausea. To keep the stomach full, recommend to your patients that they eat six small meals per day. Generally, each meal should include food sources of carbohydrate, protein, and fat.

Women should consume what appeals to them and avoid foods that cause aversion. Tolerance of specific foods with nausea and vomiting of pregnancy is highly individual. Keeping stable blood glucose levels is an additional concern. Matching rapid-acting insulin to carbohydrates consumed is useful. Some women with diabetes are able to stabilize blood glucose and intake with the use of liquid nutritional supplements, if tolerated. Other lifestyle factors, such as adequate rest and social support, may affect symptoms of nausea and vomiting. Some women may have gastroparesis and require additional individualization of the meal plan.

Table 6.1—Tips for Controlling Nausea

Remain hydrated:

- Sip fluids throughout the day (water, decaffeinated tea, ice chips)
- Maintain electrolytes, choosing lemonade, broth, diluted juice, ginger ale, popsicles, fruit ices

Avoid an empty stomach:

- Eat small frequent meals or snacks every 1–2 h
- Include protein snacks (e.g., hard-cooked eggs, nuts)
- Keep simple, dry carbohydrate foods bedside (e.g., Cheerios, saltines)
- Combine nutrients when possible, such as carbohydrate with protein (e.g., yogurt)
- Eating salty and sweet combinations is sometimes effective (e.g., lemonade and pretzels)
- Include a bedtime snack to reduce risk of early morning nausea

Avoid an overly full stomach:

- Separate intake of fluids and solid food
- Avoid large meals
- Avoid fatty foods
- Avoid foods with strong odors and flavors

Take a prenatal vitamin at dinner or bedtime

Temporarily discontinue prenatal vitamins and use a children's chewable tablet and a folic acid supplement

Anemic women should continue iron, perhaps in divided doses

Avoid caffeine

For women with hyperemesis and gastroparesis, metoclopramide is safe in pregnancy and can reduce nausea.

Caffeine also may aggravate nausea, so advise a reduction in caffeine consumption. Fried, spicy, and fatty foods increase nausea. Peppers, chilies, and garlic are often culprits. Eating certain foods, or even simply smelling their aroma, can precipitate nausea, so advise patients to avoid these foods until the morning sickness has subsided. It may help if meals can be prepared by someone else. Some clinicians suggest taking a folic acid–only supplement as this may reduce nausea compared to iron-containing prenatal vitamins.

PHARMACOLOGIC TREATMENTS

If vomiting during pregnancy is not controlled by dietary remedies, various medications may be prescribed (ACOG 2018a). Early treatment may prevent progression to severe nausea and vomiting. Pyridoxine (vitamin B_6), 10–25 mg orally every 8 h, was more effective than placebo in randomized trials (Sahakian et al. 1991, Vutyavanich et al. 1995) and is available over the counter. Doxylamine, an antihistamine, 12.5–25 mg every 8 h may be added if pyridoxine alone is unsuccessful. Doxylamine is available over the counter as a sleep aid in a 25-mg dose. Other antihistamines, such as diphenhydramine, meclizine, or dimenhydrinate, also may be prescribed. All of the antihistamines may cause drowsiness. When these approaches are not effective, prochlorperazine or promethazine may be used orally or rectally. Ondansetron 4–8 mg orally every 6 h is quite effective, and the availability of a generic version has rendered this drug less costly than in the past. Metoclopramide 10 mg every 6 h may be effective as well (Matok et al. 2009, Tan et al. 2010). It is best to recommend hospitalization if vomiting continues for 8 h, the patient has persistent hypoglycemia, or the patient has developed significant ketonuria. Treatment usually consists of intravenous (IV) fluids; potassium replacement; and close monitoring of blood glucose, urine ketones, and weight. Antiemetic medications also may be needed until the cycle of vomiting has been stopped.

For most women, symptoms generally are lessened once they have eaten and are diminished markedly by 16 weeks of gestation. Women experiencing morning sickness are statistically less likely to experience a spontaneous loss or preterm birth (Weigel and Weigel 1989). This can be especially reassuring information for women with diabetes.

INSULIN ADJUSTMENTS

The management of women with type 1 diabetes (T1D) or insulin-treated type 2 diabetes (T2D) who experience morning sickness provides a challenge for even the most skilled practitioners. Nausea may be a symptom of hypoglycemia, and hypoglycemia often aggravates nausea. It is therefore essential to have patients check their blood glucose often to avoid hypoglycemia. It is important that patients carry food at all times so that they can promptly treat any hypoglycemia or nausea. If nausea becomes severe enough to cause vomiting, women receiving insulin may need adjustments in the interval between their injection and meal-time.

The following approaches can be taken for insulin management in women with diabetes experiencing nausea and vomiting of pregnancy:

- Caution patients that they may need to decrease their short-acting insulin if they decrease their intake.
- Have patients take a portion of the insulin with a small part of the meal's carbohydrate to see how well the food is tolerated before taking the remainder of the insulin and the meal.
- Long-acting insulin (insulin glargine or insulin detemir) can be continued to prevent diabetic ketoacidosis (DKA) and hyperglycemia, even in patients with vomiting.

PRETERM BIRTH

The risk of preterm birth (birth after 20 weeks but before 37 weeks of gestation), both spontaneous and iatrogenic, appears increased in women with preexisting diabetes compared to woman who are normoglycemic (ACOG 2018b). Most reports estimate the incidence of preterm birth in women with preexisting diabetes to be between 20% and 70%, depending on type of diabetes, length of time since diagnosis, and the presence or absence of vascular complications (Jensen et al. 2010, Yanit et al. 2012, Bennett et al. 2015, Klemetti et al. 2016). These estimates are significantly higher than the general population incidence of preterm birth of 10–12% and remain consistently higher even when considering only spontaneous preterm birth. Preterm birth may be related to diabetic control, as women with spontaneous preterm delivery have higher hemoglobin A_{1c} (A1C) levels than those with term deliveries (Kovilam et al. 2002).

In general, the goal of managing preterm labor is to delay delivery for 48 h to administer antenatal corticosteroids for fetal lung maturity. Antenatal corticosteroids are recommended in women at risk for preterm birth between 23 and 37 weeks (ACOG 2016). Note that women with preexisting diabetes and gestational diabetes mellitus (GDM) were systematically excluded from the original studies of antenatal corticosteroids before 34 weeks, both because of concerns of causing maternal harm and also because of fears of unmasking randomization status as a result of the maternal hyperglycemic response to steroids. Women with GDM but not preexisting diabetes were included in the trial that suggested neonatal benefit of corticosteroids between 34 and 36 weeks (Gyamfi-Bannerman et al. 2016). The primary risk of antenatal corticosteroids is maternal hyperglycemia, which can lead to DKA or exacerbated hyperglycemia. Additionally, maternal hyperglycemia leads to fetal hyperglycemia and hyperinsulinemia, which may actually decrease, rather than increase, fetal surfactant production (Gluck and Kulovich 1973). Therefore, careful attention must be paid to maternal glycemic status when administering antenatal corticosteroids. It is estimated that hyperglycemia occurs ~24 h after the first corticosteroid dose and that, in pregnancy, a 40% increase in insulin is required to counteract the effects of corticosteroids. This estimate, however, is based on small studies, and more information is needed to guide insulin dosing in women with diabetes receiving antenatal corticosteroids (Kaushal et al. 2003, Langen et al. 2015). In most situations of preterm labor before 34 weeks, the benefits of antenatal corticosteroids outweigh the potential risks. After 34 weeks, however, antenatal steroids are routinely given to women with GDM and not to women with preexisting diabetes.

The principles of managing preterm birth are not altered by the presence of diabetes. Tocolysis may be used to administer antenatal corticosteroids. First-line tocolytic options (indomethacin and calcium channel blockers) can be used without special consideration for diabetes status.

PREECLAMPSIA

Preexisting diabetes is an independent risk factor for preeclampsia (Hanson and Persson 1993, Sibai et al. 2000), a disease characterized by hypertension and proteinuria during pregnancy (ACOG Task Force on Hypertension in Pregnancy 2013). The risk of preeclampsia increases with length of time since diagnosis: the risk of preeclampsia is ~10% in those diagnosed 10 years before pregnancy or after 20 years old, compared to 20% in those diagnosed 10–19 years before pregnancy or between the ages of 10 and 20 years old, and up to 40% in those diagnosed 20 years or more before pregnancy or before age 10 years old (Bennett et al. 2015). The presence of vascular diabetic complications (e.g., retinopathy, nephropathy, or heart disease) is associated with an up to 70% prevalence of preeclampsia.

In women with preexisting diabetes complicated by nephropathy, the diagnosis of preeclampsia can be particularly challenging. Baseline assessment (before 20 weeks) of blood pressure and renal function (i.e., serum creatinine, urine protein-to-creatinine ratio, or 24-h urine protein collection) is necessary to distinguish between preexisting disease and new-onset preeclampsia. In women with hypertension and proteinuria before pregnancy, exacerbations of hypertensive disease and worsening of proteinuria should be considered signs of preeclampsia. Practitioners, however, must be vigilant for other signs and symptoms of preeclampsia (e.g., headache, scotoma, right upper-quadrant pain, transaminitis, renal failure, oliguria, thrombocytopenia). Because preeclampsia can lead to both maternal and fetal death, overdiagnosis is often preferable to underdiagnosis.

Diabetes does not significantly alter the management of preeclampsia. Delivery remains the only cure for preeclampsia, although expectant management may be appropriate in some cases. Magnesium sulfate is used intrapartum and postpartum for seizure prophylaxis in women with preeclampsia with severe features. Dosing alterations of magnesium sulfate may be necessary in women with preexisting renal disease.

DIABETIC KETOACIDOSIS

Because of the increased insulin requirements of pregnancy, DKA develops at less severe hyperglycemic levels and patients may even be euglycemic. Risk factors for DKA include infections (influenza, urinary tract infections), insulin pump failure, treatment with antenatal corticosteroids, and patient adherence to taking medication. With aggressive diagnosis and treatment, maternal mortality is rare. Fetal mortality has improved from >33% to <10% when DKA does occur (Chauhan et al. 1996, Cullen et al. 1996).

DKA during pregnancy is diagnosed and treated in a similar fashion to that outside of pregnancy. Laboratory assessment should include pH, ketones, electrolytes, and anion gap. Treatment includes aggressive rehydration with isotonic IV fluids, IV insulin (0.2–0.4 units/kg loading dose followed by a maintenance rate), and potassium repletion.

Nonreassuring fetal heart rate tracings are very likely with maternal DKA. In most cases, the fetal tracing improves as the maternal DKA is corrected. For this reason, it is usually best to defer emergency cesarean delivery until the patient's condition has been normalized through aggressive treatment with IV fluids, insulin, and potassium. Once acid–base balance has been restored and ketosis has disappeared, the fetal heart rate tracing typically normalizes. If not, consideration can then be given to delivery for fetal indications (Montoro 2004).

CONGENITAL ANOMALIES AND PERINATAL DEATHS

Hyperglycemia in the preconception period and in the first trimester is associated with congenital anomalies. Every 1% increase in A1C is associated with a 1.7% increase in the odds of a congenital anomaly (Guerin et al. 2007). Thus, it is important that women with preexisting diabetes receive contraception and preconception counseling to avoid this teratogenic exposure and optimize both maternal and fetal health. Anomalies associated with preexisting diabetes include central nervous system malformations, neural tube defects, cardiac malformations, genitourinary malformations, and caudal regression (Sheffield et al. 2002).

The risk of miscarriage is increased in women with diabetes. Women with diabetes have a 25–44% risk of miscarriage, compared to 15% in the population that is normoglycemic (Miodovnik et al. 1984). The risk of miscarriage can be reduced to that in the population that is normoglycemic risk when glycemic targets are met (Jovanovic et al. 2005).

According to the Healthcare Quality Improvement Partnership in the U.K., the stillbirth rate for women with T1D is 8.1 per 1,000 and for women with T2D is 11.4 per 1,000. This is significantly higher than the general population rate of 4.7 per 1,000 (Healthcare Quality Improvement Partnership 2016). Most theories of the causes of increased perinatal mortality relate to maternal hyperglycemia, which leads to fetal hyperglycemia, fetal hyperinsulinemia, fetal overgrowth, fetal hypoxia, and fetal metabolic derangements. Consequently, efforts to reduce stillbirth focus largely on maternal glycemic control.

Pregnancies complicated by preexisting diabetes undergo intensive monitoring during pregnancy. Because fetal growth may be affected by diabetes, and because fetal over- and undergrowth is strongly associated with perinatal mortality in diabetes, women undergo serial ultrasounds for fetal growth (typically every 4 weeks after 28 weeks). Additionally, at least weekly antenatal testing is recommended; twice weekly testing is frequently used in patients with diabetes, particularly those with poor glycemic control, large-for-gestational-age fetuses, or polyhydramnios. In the U.S., antenatal testing typically starts after 32 weeks of gestation. Antenatal testing may be in the form of a nonstress test, contraction stress test, modified biophysical profile, or biophysical profile, and depends largely on availability and provider preference. The risk of stillbirth for 7 days after a reassuring antenatal test is between 0.5 and 1.2 per 1,000.

Delivery timing to reduce stillbirth has not been well defined. For uncomplicated pregnancies, delivery before 39 weeks is not recommended because of the risk of respiratory distress and significant neonatal morbidity (ACOG 2018b). Because of the increased risk of stillbirth, pregnancies complicated by diabetes may require late preterm or early term delivery (34–39 weeks) (Spong et al. 2011, ACOG 2018b). The exact timing depends on maternal glycemia, diabetes history, maternal comorbidities, antenatal testing, and fetal growth.

REFERENCES

American College of Obstetricians and Gynecologists. Practice bulletin no. 171: Management of preterm labor. *Obstet Gynecol* 2016;128(4):e155–e164

American College of Obstetricians and Gynecologists. Practice bulletin no. 198: Nausea and vomiting of pregnancy. *Obstet Gynecol* 2018a;131(1):e15–e30

American College of Obstetricians and Gynecologists. Practice bulletin no. 201: Pregestational diabetes mellitus. *Obstet Gynecol* 2018b;132(6):e228–e248

American College of Obstetricians and Gynecologists, Task Force on Hypertension in Pregnancy. Hypertension in pregnancy. Report of the American College of Obstetricians and Gynecologists' Task Force on Hypertension in Pregnancy. *Obstet Gynecol* 2013;122(5):1122–1131

Bennett SN, Tita A, Owen J, Biggio JR, Harper LM. Assessing White's classification of pregestational diabetes in a contemporary diabetic population. *Obstet Gynecol* 2015;125(5):1217–1223

Borrelli F, Capasso R, Aviello G, Pittler MH, Izzo AA. Effectiveness and safety of ginger in the treatment of pregnancy-induced nausea and vomiting. *Obstet Gynecol* 2005;105:849–856

Buckwalter JG, Simpson SW. Psychological factors in the etiology and treatment of severe nausea and vomiting in pregnancy. *Am J Obstet Gynecol* 2002;186: s210–s214

Chauhan SP, Perry KG, Jr., McLaughlin BN, Roberts WE, Sullivan CA, Morrison JC. Diabetic ketoacidosis complicating pregnancy. *J Perinatol* 1996; 16(3 Pt. 1):173–175

Cullen MT, Reece EA, Homko CJ, Sivan E. The changing presentations of diabetic ketoacidosis during pregnancy. *Am J Perinatol* 1996;13(7):449–451

Czeizel AE, Dudas I, Fritz G, Tecsoi A, Hanck A, Kunovitz G. The effect of periconceptional multivitamin-mineral supplementation on vertigo, nausea and vomiting in the first trimester of pregnancy. *Arch Gynecol Obstet* 1992;251:181–185

Emelianova S, Mazzotta P, Einarson A, Koren G. Prevalence and severity of nausea and vomiting of pregnancy and effect of vitamin supplementation. *Clin Invest Med* 1999;22:106–110

Gluck L, Kulovich MV. Lecithin/sphingomyelin ratios in amniotic fluid in normal and abnormal pregnancies. *Am J Obstet Gynecol* 1973;115:64–70

Guerin A, Nisenbaum R, Ray JG. Use of maternal GHb concentration to estimate the risk of congenital anomalies in the offspring of women with prepregnancy diabetes. *Diabetes Care* 2007;30(7):1920–1925

Gyamfi-Bannerman C, Thom EA, Blackwell SC, et al. Antenatal betamethasone for women at risk for late preterm delivery. *N Engl J Med* 2016;374: 1311–1320

Hanson U, Persson B. Outcome of pregnancies complicated by type 1 insulin-dependent diabetes in Sweden: acute pregnancy complications, neonatal mortality and morbidity. *Am J Perinatol* 1993;10(4):330–333

Healthcare Quality Improvement Partnership. National Pregnancy in Diabetes 2015. Published 21 October 2016. Available from www.hqip.org.uk/wp-content/uploads/2018/02/summary-national-pregnancy-in-diabetes-2015.pdf. Accessed 24 February 2019

Jensen DM, Damm P, Ovesen P, Molsted-Pedersen L, Beck-Nielsen H, Wester-gaard JG, Moeller M, Mathiesen ER. Microalbuminuria, preeclampsia, and preterm delivery in pregnant women with type 1 diabetes: results from a nationwide Danish study. *Diabetes Care* 2010;33(1):90–94

Jovanovic L, Knopp RH, Kim H, Cefalu WT, Zhu XD, Lee YJ, Simpson JL, Mills JL. Elevated pregnancy losses at high and low extremes of maternal glucose in early normal and diabetic pregnancy: evidence for a protective adaptation in diabetes. *Diabetes Care* 2005;28(5):1113–1117

Kaushal K, Gibson JM, Railton A, Hounsome B, New JP, Young RJ. A protocol for improved glycaemic control following corticosteroid therapy in diabetic pregnancies. *Diabet Med* 2003;20(1):73–75

Klemetti MM, Laivuori H, Tikkanen M, Nuutila M, Hiilesmaa V, Teramo K. White's classification and pregnancy outcome in women with type 1 diabetes: a population-based cohort study. *Diabetologia* 2016;59(1):92–100

Kovilam O, Khoury J, Miodovnik M, Chames M, Spinnoto J, Sibai B. Spontaneous preterm delivery in the type 1 diabetic pregnancy: the role of glycemic control. *J Matern Fetal Neonatal Med* 2002;11(4):245–248

Langen ES, Kuperstock JL, Sung JF, Taslimi M, Byrne J, El-Sayed YY. Maternal glucose response to betamethasone administration. *Am J Perinatol* 2015;30(2):143–148

Matok I, Gorodischer R, Koren G, Sheiner E, Wiznitzer A, Levy A. The safety of metoclopramide use in the first trimester of pregnancy. *N Engl J Med* 2009;360:2528–2535

Miodovnik M, Lavin JP, Knowles HC, Holroyde J, Stys SJ. Spontaneous abortion among insulin-dependent diabetic women. *Am J Obstet Gynecol* 1984;150(4):372–376

Montoro MM. Diabetic ketoacidosis in pregnancy. In *Diabetes in Women: Adolescence, Pregnancy, and Menopause*. Reece EA, Coustan DR, Gabbe SG, Eds. Philadelphia, PA, Lippincott Williams & Wilkins, 2004, p. 345–350

Sahakian V, Rouse D, Sipes S, Rose N, Niebyl J. Vitamin B6 is effective therapy for nausea and vomiting of pregnancy: a randomized, double-blind placebo-controlled study. *Obstet Gynecol* 1991;78:33–36

Sheffield JS, Butler-Koster EL, Casey BM, McIntire DD, Leveno KJ. Maternal diabetes mellitus and infant malformations. *Obstet Gynecol* 2002;100(5 Pt 1):925–930

Sibai BM, Caritis S, Hauth J, Lindheimer M, VanDorsten JP, MacPherson C, Klebanoff M, Landon M, Miodovnik M, Paul R, Meis P, Dombrowski M, Thurnau G, Roberts J, McNellis D. Risks of preeclampsia and adverse neonatal outcomes among women with pregestational diabetes mellitus. National Institute of Child Health and Human Development Network of Maternal-Fetal Medicine Units. *Am J Obstet Gynecol* 2000;182(2):364–369

Spong CY, Mercer BM, D'Alton M, Kilpatrick S, Blackwell S, Saade G. Timing of indicated late-preterm and early-term birth. *Obstet Gynecol* 2011;118 (2 Pt. 1):323–333

Tan PC, Jacob R, Quek KF, Omar SZ. The fetal sex ratio and metabolic, biochemical, haematological and clinical indicators of severity of hyperemesis gravidarum. *Br J Obstet Gynaecol* 2006;113:733–737

Tan PC, Khine PP, Vallikkannu N, Omar SZ. Promethazine compared with metoclopramide for hyperemesis gravidarum: a randomized controlled trial. *Obstet Gynecol* 2010;115:975–981

Vutyavanich T, Wongtra-ngan S, Ruangsri R. Pyridoxine for nausea and vomiting of pregnancy: a randomized, double-blind, placebo-controlled trial. *Am J Obstet Gynecol* 1995;173:881–884

Weigel MM, Weigel RM. Nausea and vomiting of early pregnancy and pregnancy outcome: an epidemiological study. *Br J Obstet Gynaecol* 1989;96:1304–1311

Yanit KE, Snowden JM, Cheng YW, Caughey AB. The impact of chronic hypertension and pregestational diabetes on pregnancy outcomes. *Am J Obstet Gynecol* 2012;207(4):333.e331–336

Neonatal Care of Infants of Mothers with Diabetes

Highlights
Neonatal Care of Infants of
Mothers with Diabetes

■ Although many infants of mothers with diabetes have an uneventful perinatal course, there is still an increased rate of complications.

■ Of factors influencing neonatal morbidity in pregnancies affected by diabetes, the most significant single factor is the gestational age of the pregnancy.

■ Maintenance of a normal metabolic state, including euglycemia, should diminish but will not eradicate the increased potential for perinatal and neonatal morbidities.

■ Women with diabetes optimally should be delivered in tertiary care centers with specialized management.

■ Neonatal resuscitation requires a fully equipped area and knowledgeable personnel. Evaluation of the neonate should include observation for macrosomia, birth injury, avoidance of asphyxia, presence of congenital malformations, respiratory distress, and hypoglycemia.

■ Nursery care of the infant can be accomplished in a regular nursery or special-care unit, if one exists in the delivery hospital, depending on the infant's gestational age and the presence or absence of morbidities. The more appropriate the birth weight relative to the gestational age of the infant, the greater chance for care in a regular nursery.

Neonatal Care of Infants of Mothers with Diabetes

The infant of the mother with diabetes exemplifies the morbidities that may exist in the neonate because of maternal disease (Cowett 1991a). Developmentally, neonates are in a transitional state of glucose homeostasis. The fetus is completely dependent on the mother for glucose transfer in utero, and maintenance of glucose homeostasis may be a significant problem. The neonate must maintain a balance between glucose deficiency and excess. The dependence of the conceptus on the mother for continuous substrate delivery contrasts with the variable and intermittent exogenous oral intake by the neonate. Development of homeostasis results from a balance between substrate availability and developmental hormonal, sympathomimetic, and enzymatic systems (Cowett 1991b). The precarious nature of this balance is reinforced by the numerous morbidities associated with altered states of neonatal glucose homeostasis. This chapter highlights specific factors that are important in the immediate care of the infants born to women with diabetes in the delivery room and their subsequent care both in the nursery and after discharge from the hospital.

OVERVIEW

The physician responsible for the care and delivery of the mother should inform the physician responsible for the care of the neonate well in advance of delivery. Factors of importance include the following:

- Knowledge of the character of the maternal diabetes (including diabetes type, glycemia, and blood pressure control)
- Prior pregnancy history
- Complications occurring during the pregnancy (including results of fetal ultrasounds, episodes of maternal infection, vaginal bleeding, and medications administered)

Knowing these facts allows the physician caring for the neonate to anticipate many of the potential fetal and neonatal complications. These factors determine whether a pediatric provider or neonatologist needs to be present at delivery, although in many institutions delivery of a mother with diabetes always will have pediatric personnel in attendance.

Hanson et al. (1986) evaluated factors influencing neonatal morbidity in pregnancies affected by diabetes. In 92 consecutive pregnancies, those with severe morbidity had the following:

- Longer duration of maternal diabetes
- Shorter gestational age at birth
- Higher rates of cesarean delivery
- Higher frequency of preeclampsia

The most significant single factor was the gestational age of the pregnancy. In this study, maternal glucose control between 70 and 153 mg/dL (3.8 and 8.5 mmol/L) during pregnancy and in labor did not significantly influence morbidity. Thus, the maintenance of a normal metabolic state likely improves outcomes by lengthening gestation, but it will not completely eradicate the increased perinatal and neonatal mortality and morbidities of pregnancies affected by diabetes.

A more recent study showed that neonates were ~48 g heavier at birth for each 18 mg/dL increase in maternal glycemia above euglycemia in 4,681 pregnancies (Stenhouse et al. 2006). With an increase in birth weight, there also was an increased risk of complications in the neonatal period. Maternal diabetes remains the major independent risk factor for fetal macrosomia. Rates of congenital anomalies are also two to five times higher in women with preexisting diabetes than the rates in infants born to women without diabetes, and these rates have not changed over the past 20 years (Wyatt et al. 2004). Thus, the neonatologist must be aware that the newborn of a woman with diabetes should be treated as high risk until proven otherwise.

NEWBORN OUTCOMES

CONGENITAL ANOMALIES

Although most of the morbidity and mortality data for infants born to women with diabetes show improvement with advances in the care of the mothers during pregnancy, congenital anomalies remain a major unresolved problem. The two- to fivefold increase in the incidence of congenital anomalies has been long noted in most centers and remains a frequent contributor to perinatal mortality (Miller et al. 1981, Ballard et al. 1984, Goldman 1986, Schwartz and Teramo 2000, Sheffield et al. 2002, Wren et al. 2003, Touger et al. 2005, Hay 2012; Table 7.1).

Table 7.1—Discrete Patterns of Congenital Anomalies in Infants of Mothers with Diabetes

- Major congenital heart disease
- Musculoskeletal deformities, including caudal regression syndrome
- Central nervous system deformities (anencephaly, spina bifida, hydrocephalus)
- Genitourinary anomalies
- Gastrointestinal abnormalities

The prevalence and spectrum of cardiovascular anomalies in infants born to mothers with preexisting diabetes compared with those in infants of mothers without diabetes have been assessed prospectively in a geographic region of the U.K. between 1995 and 2000 (Wren et al. 2003). There were 192,618 live births; cardiovascular malformations occurred in 3.6% of infants of pregnancies affected by diabetes and in 0.74% of infants of pregnancies not affected by diabetes (odds ratio [OR] 5.0; 95% confidence interval [CI] 3.3–7.8). There was a more than threefold increase in transposition of the great vessels, truncus arteriosus, and tricuspid atresia among infants born to mothers with diabetes.

The pathogenesis of the increased frequency of congenital anomalies among the infants born to women with diabetes remains obscure (Touger et al. 2005). Several etiologies have been proposed to account for the incidence of anomalies:

- Hyperglycemia, either preconceptional or postconceptional
- Hypoglycemia
- Uteroplacental vascular disease
- Genetic predisposition

Although there are data to support each proposal, the evidence is best for the preconceptional and early postconceptional hyperglycemia etiology (Kitzmiller et al. 1978, Miller et al. 1981, Fuhrmann et al. 1983, Ballard et al. 1984, Goldman et al. 1986, Freinkel et al. 1990, Metzger and Buchanan 1990). The preponderance of evidence indicates that early rigid glucose control will minimize the incidence of anomalies (Schwartz and Teramo 2000). A study of 145,196 women, for example, showed that women with preexisting diabetes or gestational diabetes plus fasting hyperglycemia have a three- to fourfold increased risk of congenital anomalies, whereas women with gestational diabetes mellitus (GDM) without fasting hyperglycemia had malformation rates similar to the general obstetric population without diabetes (Sheffield et al. 2002). The critical period of teratogenesis occurs before the 7th week postconception. In contrast, poor glucose control later in pregnancy carries a higher risk of macrosomia, intrauterine growth restriction, asphyxia, and fetal death (Hay 2012).

CARDIOMYOPATHY

Hypertrophic cardiomyopathy observed in the infants born to women with diabetes primarily affects the interventricular septum and, to a smaller degree, the ventricular free walls (Hornberger 2006). It can be present irrespective of reasonable metabolic control (Hornberger 2006). Respiratory distress can be accompanied by septal hypertrophy (Way et al. 1979, Reller and Kaplan 1988), with resolution of symptoms within 2–4 weeks and of the hypertrophy within 2–12 months (Mace et al. 1979). Hypertrophy of the interventricular septum and walls of the right and left ventricles also has been documented (Breitweser et al. 1980). Profound hypoglycemia after birth, consistent with the metabolic effects of neonatal hyperinsulinism, has been strongly associated with septal hypertrophy (Ballard et al. 1984). Fetal hyperinsulinism may contribute directly to septal hypertrophy.

Although cardiac hypertrophy, apart from congenital heart disease, has been recognized in autopsies of infants born to women with diabetes, it is now understood that some infants have a peculiar form of subaortic stenosis similar to the idiopathic hypertrophic subaortic stenosis found in adults (Halliday 1981). This particular entity may be associated with symptomatic congestive heart failure. As with the adult variant, in these neonates, therapy with digoxin is contraindicated because the resultant increased myocardial contractility has been reported to be deleterious. Propranolol appears to be the therapeutic drug of choice. Clinically, this disorder resolves spontaneously over a period of weeks to months with a correction of the echocardiographic features as well.

MACROSOMIA, BIRTH INJURY, AND ASPHYXIA

The neonates of women not achieving glucose targets often will appear macrosomic (>4 kg [>8 lb, 13 oz] at term or >90th percentile in weight for gestational age) in contrast to neonates of women who are meeting glycemic targets and women who do not have diabetes or obesity (Cowett 1991a). The incidence of macrosomia increases significantly as the mean maternal blood glucose concentrations exceed 130 mg/dL in the third trimester (Hay 2012). A consequence of undetected fetal macrosomia may be a difficult vaginal delivery, including shoulder dystocia and birth injury or asphyxia (Table 7.2).

Table 7.2—Potential Birth Injuries in Infants of Mothers with Diabetes

- Brachial plexus injury
- Abdominal organ injury
- Facial palsy
- Cephalohematoma
- Ocular hemorrhage
- Clavicular fracture
- Subdural hemorrhage
- Diaphragmatic paralysis
- External genitalia hemorrhage

Injury to the brachial plexus may appear with a variety of presentations because the nerves of the brachial plexus may be damaged. In addition to the obvious injury to the nerves of the arm, diaphragmatic paralysis occurs if the phrenic nerve is affected. Because of the associated organomegaly in some infants born to women with diabetes, hemorrhage in the abdominal organs is possible, specifically in the liver and adrenal glands. Hemorrhage in the external genitalia of large neonates has been noted.

Because these neonates are at high risk, intrapartum monitoring may reduce potential complications. At delivery, the nursing personnel evaluating the neonate assign Apgar scores at 1 and 5 min to document the adequacy of transition from in utero to extrauterine existence. Although there are many reasons for poor transition among neonates born to women with diabetes, relative macrosomia may predispose the fetus and newborn to fetal acidemia. Thus, a cord pH provides an easily obtainable early biochemical assessment of the fetus.

Asphyxia may complicate delivery in pregnancies affected by diabetes and can result in multiorgan dysfunction. It may affect respiratory, renal, and central nervous system (CNS) functions acutely and also may result in hematological (thrombocytopenia, disseminated intravascular coagulation), metabolic (syndrome of inappropriate antidiuretic hormone secretion, hypocalcemia), myocardial, and hepatic abnormalities. Stabilization of altered hemodynamics (hypotension, poor perfusion, acidemia) is a priority followed by decreased fluid intake because of the potential for renal and CNS injury.

INTRAUTERINE GROWTH RESTRICTION

Intrauterine growth restriction can occur if maternal diabetes is associated with severe vascular disease (defined as the presence of at least one of the following: diabetic retinopathy, diabetic nephropathy, or preexisting hypertension) (Gutaj 2016). This is particularly the case among women with type 1 diabetes (T1D) who experience frequent hypo- and hyperglycemia. Such pregnancies should have intensive fetal monitoring to detect the safest time for delivery (Gutaj 2016).

RESPIRATORY DISTRESS

Respiratory distress, including respiratory distress syndrome (RDS), used to be a frequent and potentially severe complication of preexisting diabetes. Improved management of blood glucose levels and modern obstetric management in the setting of preterm birth, including administration of antenatal steroids, have greatly reduced the incidence of RDS. Neonatal RDS (pathologic correlate: hyaline membrane disease) develops because of lung immaturity in the neonate and remains a major cause of mortality. Other causes of respiratory distress in the infant born to a woman with diabetes exist as well (Table 7.3).

Table 7.3—Causes of Respiratory Distress in Infants of Mothers with Diabetes, Other Than Respiratory Distress Syndrome

- Cardiac disease
- Transient tachypnea
- Diaphragmatic hernia
- Pneumothorax
- Meconium aspiration

RDS has a typical course that is manifested by increasing oxygen requirements as a result of progressive respiratory compromise. Tachypnea, intercostal and subcostal retractions, nasal flaring, and expiratory grunting appearing in the first few minutes to hours of life are the cardinal signs of the disease. In uncomplicated cases, the disease usually peaks by 72 h of age. With the use of exogenous surfactant, the time course of RDS has been shortened significantly for the majority of infants. Complications commonly associated with RDS include air leaks (the latter has been reduced by surfactant), the presence of a persistent patent ductus arteriosus in preterm infants, and bronchopulmonary dysplasia in preterm infants requiring prolonged ventilatory support and high ambient oxygen concentrations. Both of these conditions may significantly lengthen the clinical course of an otherwise self-limited disease. RDS should be managed with particular attention to the following:

- Fluid administration and avoiding unneeded volume expansion
- Supplemental oxygen
- Continuous positive airway pressure
- Ventilator support when necessary
- Exogenous surfactant if intubation is needed

HYPOGLYCEMIA

A rapid decrease in neonatal plasma glucose concentration after delivery is characteristic after a pregnancy complicated by diabetes. The blood or plasma glucose concentration that is thought to be abnormal continues to be debated among care providers (Adamkin 2011). For many practitioners, however, values <35 mg/dL (<1.9 mmol/L) in term infants are considered abnormal and may occur within 30 min following clamping of the umbilical cord (Srinivasan et al. 1986). Factors that may influence the degree of hypoglycemia include previous maternal glucose homeostasis and maternal glycemia during labor and delivery (Cowett 1991b). A patient not meeting glycemic targets will result in stimulating the fetal pancreas leading to excessive insulin release. Neonatal hypoglycemia may persist for 48 h or may develop after 24 h (Lin et al. 1989). The neonate exhibits transitional control of glucose metabolism, which suggests that a multiplicity of factors affect homeostasis. Many of the factors are similar to those that influence homeostasis in the adult. There is blunted splanchnic (hepatic) responsiveness to insulin in both the preterm and term neonate, however, compared with the adult (Cowett 1988a).

HYPOCALCEMIA AND HYPOMAGNESEMIA

In addition to hypoglycemia, hypocalcemia (defined as a total serum calcium concentration <7 mg/dL) ranks as an important metabolic derangement observed in neonates born to women with diabetes (Schwartz and Teramo 2000). During pregnancy, fetal calcium needs increase maternal calcium demands. Usually, an increase in maternal calcium absorption from the gut supplies the needed calcium. This increase in calcium absorption seems to be mediated by an increase in maternal 1,25-dihydroxyvitamin D. The increase in 1,25-dihydroxyvitamin D occurs despite the parathyroid hormone levels being in the low-normal range throughout gestation and likely is due to the increased production of 1,25-dihydroxyvitamin D by the kidneys and the fetoplacental unit (Cooper 2011).

In a case series of 532 infants born to 332 women with gestational diabetes and 177 women with preexisting diabetes, hypoglycemia occurred in 27% of infants and hypocalcemia was documented in only 4% of infants. Low rates of hypocalcemia are speculated to reflect glycemic targets being met during pregnancy and the appropriate triage of infants in anticipation of neonatal problems (Cordero et al. 1998).

Hypomagnesemia (<1.5 mg/dL) also may occur in neonates born to women with diabetes, often in association with hypocalcemia. As with hypocalcemia, the frequency and severity of clinical symptoms are correlated with maternal status. Neonatal magnesium concentration has been correlated with that in the mother as well as with the maternal insulin requirements and concentration of intravenous glucose administered to the neonate (Noguchi et al. 1980). Although the exact cause of hypocalcemia is not well understood, it may be secondary to decreased parathyroid function and hypomagnesia in the infant (Cruikshank et al. 1983). Hypocalcemia and hypomagnesemia may have clinical manifestations similar to those of hypoglycemia in addition to those of tetany and should be treated accordingly.

HYPERBILIRUBINEMIA AND ERYTHREMIA

Hyperbilirubinemia is observed more frequently in neonates born to women with GDM or preexisting diabetes. The pathogenesis remains uncertain (Cowett 1988b, 1991a; Yang et al. 2006). Prematurity (biochemical immaturity) has been rejected as an explanation (Burns et al. 2008). Other etiologies of hyperbilirubinemia have been related to hemolysis with decreased erythrocyte survival. However, erythrocyte life span, osmotic fragility, and deformability have not been found to be appreciably different in neonates born to women with preexisting diabetes or GDM compared to women with euglycemia (Taylor et al. 1963, Peevy et al. 1980). Delayed clearance of the bilirubin load, however, measured by pulmonary excretion of carbon monoxide as an index of bilirubin production, may be a factor (Stevenson et al. 1981a, 1981b).

The erythremia (polycythemia is a misnomer, because only the erythrocyte mass is elevated, not the leukocyte count or the platelet count) frequently observed in infants born to women with diabetes may be the most important factor associated with hyperbilirubinemia. Venous hematocrits of 65–70% have been observed in 20–40% of infants born to women with diabetes during the first days of life, and sometimes have been associated with signs and symptoms of neonatal erythremia, such as jitteriness, seizures, tachypnea, priapism, and oliguria (Salvesen et al. 1992). Therapy with the use of a partial-exchange transfusion (10–15% of total blood volume) through the umbilical vein with normal saline or 5% albumin has been associated with a rapid resolution of symptoms.

NURSERY CARE

The presence of the specific morbidities discussed thus far requires specialized attention by care providers who have the knowledge, training, and experience. Given this consideration, the clinician should decide whether to observe the infant born to a woman with preexisting diabetes or GDM in a special-care nursery or follow the neonate in the regular nursery, assuming both exist in the delivering hospital, or transfer the infant to a special-care unit at another health center (Table 7.4). Even if the infant can be cared for in the regular nursery, specific metabolic abnormalities should be looked for, including the following:

- Hypoglycemia
- Hypocalcemia
- Hypomagnesemia
- Erythremia
- Hyperbilirubinemia

Table 7.4—Factors Indicating That the Infant of a Mother with Diabetes Will Need Care in a Special-Care Nursery

- Asphyxia
- Birth injury
- Congenital anomalies
- Hypoglycemia
- Tetany
- Large or small for gestational age

GLUCOSE HOMEOSTASIS

All infants are at risk for abnormal glucose hemostasis in the newborn period, and this risk is accentuated in infants of pregnancies affected by diabetes. Similar to infants of pregnancies not affected by diabetes, infants of mothers with diabetes can appear asymptomatic even with a relatively low plasma glucose concentration. This may be due to the initial brain stores of glycogen; other etiologies include the use of alternative substrates for oxidative metabolism because concentrations of lactate and ketone bodies frequently are elevated shortly after birth.

Although a laboratory determination of blood glucose is the most accurate method, it does not provide results in real time, which are needed for screening for hypoglycemia. Bedside reagent test-strip glucose analyzers can be used if the test is performed with proper quality control measures and if providers are aware of the limitations of such devices (Adamkin 2011). In view of the limitations of bedside rapid determinations of blood glucose concentration, abnormal values should be confirmed with stat laboratory testing. Neonates may require parenteral treatment for maintenance of carbohydrate homeostasis. Early administration of oral feeding shortly after birth may be beneficial to maintain plasma glucose concentrations that are not depressed.

The neonate who has a glucose concentration <40 mg/dL (<2.2 mmol/L) at ≤4 h of age (for both the term and preterm neonate) in the presence of symptoms (see Table 7.5) should be treated with glucose administered intravenously.

Bolus injection without subsequent infusion will only exaggerate the hypoglycemia by a rebound mechanism and is contraindicated. Minibolus therapy (200 mg/kg or 2 cc/kg of 10% dextrose) has been demonstrated to avoid rebound hypoglycemia (Lilien et al. 1980) and can be followed with infusion of 6–8 mg/kg/min of glucose. Once plasma glucose stabilizes to >45 mg/dL (>2.5 mmol/L), the infusion may be slowly decreased while oral feedings are initiated and advanced. If symptomatic hypoglycemia persists, higher glucose rates of ≥8–12 mg/kg/min may be necessary and may necessitate insertion of an umbilical venous catheter to use higher dextrose concentrations and to avoid excessive fluid administration. Because most neonates are asymptomatic, glucagon administration to prevent hypoglycemia after delivery does not appear warranted. Furthermore, glucagon may stimulate insulin release, which may exaggerate the tendency for hypoglycemia.

Table 7.5—Signs and Symptoms of Neonatal Hypoglycemia

Abnormal cry	Convulsions	Jitteriness
Apathy	Cyanosis	Lethargy
Apnea	Hypothermia	Tremors
Cardiac arrest	Hypotonia	Tachypnea

Prompt recognition and treatment of neonatal hypoglycemia has minimized sequelae. Glucose is the principal substrate for cerebral metabolism, and hypoglycemia can cause neuronal and glial injury (Banker 1967, Koivisto et al. 1972). The independent effect of hypoglycemia, however, is difficult to determine in the clinical setting. In prospective evaluations of low–birth weight infants, moderate hypoglycemia (<2.6 mmol/L) has been associated with an increase in neurodevelopmental sequelae (Lucas et al. 1988). With the use of magnetic resonance imaging (MRI), the effect of hypoglycemia has been investigated in more recent cohorts of infants to determine whether a specific neurologic pattern of injury can be observed in infants who experienced symptomatic neonatal hypoglycemia (Karimzadeh et al. 2011). Ninety percent of infants showed abnormal signal in the posterior cerebral area supporting a hypoglycemia-occipital syndrome. Others have also reported an association between neonatal hypoglycemia and occipital cerebral injury with links to long-term disability, epilepsy, and visual impairment (Filan et al. 2006). Not all reports, however, have confirmed these associations. In a cohort of 35 term infants with symptomatic neonatal hypoglycemia (median glucose level of 1 mmol/L) without evidence of hypoxic-ischemic encephalopathy, patterns of injury on MRI were varied with white-matter abnormalities being the most common (94%); a predominant posterior pattern occurred in only 29% of cases (Burns et al. 2008). Twenty-three infants (65%) demonstrated impairments at 18 months that were related to the severity of the white-matter injury and not to the location (Burns et al. 2008). These studies confirm the potential for symptomatic hypoglycemia to be associated with brain injury.

RESUSCITATION

As with any neonate who is considered high risk immediately after delivery, neonates born after a pregnancy complicated by diabetes requiring resuscitation and stabilization should be taken care of in a designated resuscitation area. As noted by the *Guidelines for Perinatal Care* (American Academy of Pediatrics and the American College of Obstetricians and Gynecologists [AAP/ACOG] 2017), resuscitation should be carried out in a fully equipped area illuminated to at least 100 foot-candles and containing equipment required for skilled resuscitation (Table 7.6). A more detailed accounting can be obtained from the AAP/ACOG guidelines (2017). Likewise, specific personnel should be available, dedicated to devoting their complete attention to the neonate. The American Heart Association and American Academy of Pediatrics have produced materials to teach resuscitation skills (AAP 2016, AAP/ACOG 2017). All neonates need to be dried off initially to maintain as close to a neutral thermal environment as possible. Evaluation of the infant in the resuscitation room requires observation for multiple factors (Table 7.7).

Table 7.6—Equipment Required in Resuscitation

- An overhead source of radiant heat that can be regulated relative to the neonate's body temperature
- Airway stabilization equipment (devices to provide positive pressure ventilation, laryngoscope, endotracheal tube, etc.)
- Pulse oximeter, oxygen, compressed air, and suction dedicated to the neonate
- Trays with medications, fluids (epinephrine, normal saline)
- Wall clock
- Charting surface
- Catheters, needles, stopcocks, infusion pumps

Table 7.7—Elements to Be Evaluated in the Resuscitation Room for Infants Born to Mothers with Diabetes

- Poor respiratory effort
- Birth injury
- Congenital anomalies
- Erythremia
- Evidence of macrosomia
- Respiratory distress

OFFSPRING ADIPOSITY AND CARDIOMETABOLIC HEALTH

Studies examining the association between maternal diabetes and offspring adiposity have been conflicting. A meta-analysis reported that the evidence supporting an association between maternal diabetes and greater offspring body mass index (BMI) is still inconclusive (Philipps et al. 2011). Although there was a positive association between gestational and preexisting diabetes in pregnancy and offspring adiposity, this association was attenuated after adjusting for maternal prepregnancy BMI (Philipps et al. 2011). Separate studies also confirmed that childhood obesity at 2–4 years of age was not associated with GDM but was associated with maternal BMI (Pham et al. 2013). Yet another meta-analysis showed that maternal diabetes was still significantly associated with higher fat mass in infancy even after adjusting for maternal prepregnancy BMI (Logan et al. 2017). Family studies are also supportive of an association between maternal diabetes and offspring adiposity. For example, among the Pima Indians of central Arizona, a population with a very high prevalence of type 2 diabetes (T2D), offspring born to mothers with T2D had greater mean BMI, increased fasting glucose and insulin, and higher risk of developing T2D at an early age than offspring born before the mother was diagnosed with diabetes (Dabelea et al. 2000, Pettitt et al. 1993). The risk of diabetes was more than threefold (OR 3.7; 95% CI 1.3–11.3) among siblings born after the mother developed diabetes than among those born before the mother's diabetes diagnosis (Dabelea et al. 2000). Studies also indicate higher systolic blood pressure (Aceti et al. 2012) and a higher rate of the metabolic syndrome among offspring of mothers with diabetes. The development of the metabolic syndrome (obesity, hypertension, dyslipidemia, and glucose intolerance) has been examined among large-for-gestation and appropriate-for-gestation offspring of mothers with or without GDM at ages 6–11 years old (Boney et al. 2005). Large-for-gestational-age offspring of mothers with diabetes were at significant risk of developing metabolic syndrome in childhood (hazard ratio 2.19; 95% CI 1.25–3.82) (Boney et al. 2005). Furthermore, adult offspring of women with diet-treated GDM and T1D appear to be at risk for obesity and the metabolic syndrome (Clausen et al. 2009).

OFFSPRING COGNITIVE ABILITIES

Few studies are available examining the associations between diabetes in pregnancy and offspring's cognitive development. A systematic review examined 14 articles addressing the cognitive development of offspring (age ≤12 years) as outcome and any diabetes in pregnancy as exposure (Adane et al. 2016). Of the 14 articles, 10 studies investigated the associations between maternal preexisting diabetes or both preexisting diabetes and GDM and offspring's cognitive development with six studies reporting at least one negative association (Adane et al. 2016). The other four studies examined the relationships between GDM only and offspring's cognitive development with two studies reporting a negative association, one a positive association, and one a null association (Adane et al. 2016). The inconsistent findings among these studies might be due to limited statistical power, study population differences, utilizing different measures of cognitive ability, and adjustment for potential confounders such as prepregnancy obesity and maternal socioeconomic status (Adane et al. 2016). Other studies, including a large Swedish record-linkage study of 6,397 offspring of mothers with diabetes in pregnancy, reported that maternal diabetes in pregnancy was associated with a greater risk of not completing compulsory schooling at the age of 16 years (OR 1.25; 95% CI 1.10–1.43) and with a lower average school mark (Dahlquist and Kallen 2007). In a cohort of Danish women, offspring of women with T1D were reported to have lower standardized intelligence indices at 13–19 years old compared with controls (Bytoft et al. 2016).

REFERENCES

Aceti A, Santhakumaran S, Logan KM, Philipps LH, Prior E, Gale C, Hyde MJ, Modi N. The diabetic pregnancy and offspring blood pressure in childhood: a systematic review and meta-analysis. *Diabetologia* 2012;55:3114–3127

Adamkin DH, Committee on Fetus and Newborn. Postnatal glucose homeostasis in late preterm and term infants. *Pediatrics* 2011;127:575–579

Adane AA, Mishra GD, Tooth LR. Diabetes in pregnancy and childhood cognitive development: a systematic review. *Pediatrics* 2016;137:e20154234

American Academy of Pediatrics. *Textbook of Neonatal Resuscitation.* 7th ed. Dallas, TX, American Heart Association, 2016

American Academy of Pediatrics and the American College of Obstetricians and Gynecologists. *Guidelines for Perinatal Care.* 8th ed. Kilpatrick SJ, Papile LA, Eds. Washington, DC, American Academy of Pediatrics, 2017

Ballard J, Holroyde J, Tsang RC, Chan G, Sutherland JM, Knowles HC. High malformation rates and decreased mortality in infants of diabetic mothers managed after the first trimester (1956–1978). *Am J Obstet Gynecol* 1984;148: 111–118

Banker BQ. The neuropathological effects of anoxia and hypoglycemia in the newborn. *Dev Med Child Neurol* 1967;9:544–550

Boney CM, Verma A, Tucker R, Vohr BR. Metabolic syndrome in childhood: association with birth weight, maternal obesity and gestational diabetes mellitus. *Pediatrics* 2005;115:e290–e296

Breitweser JA, Mayer RA, Sperling MA, Psang RC, Kaplan S. Cardiac septal hypertrophy in hyperinsulinemic infants. *J Pediatr* 1980;96:535–539

Burns CM, Rutherford MA, Boardman JP, Cowan FM. Patterns of cerebral injury and neurodevelopmental outcomes after symptomatic neonatal hypoglycemia. *Pediatrics* 2008;122:65–74

Bytoft B, Knorr S, Vlachova Z, Jensen RB, Mathiesen ER, Beck-Nielsen H, Gravholt CH, Jensen DM, Clausen TD, Mortensen EL, Damm P. Long-term cognitive implications of intrauterine hyperglycemia in adolescent offspring of women with type 1 diabetes (the EPICOM Study). *Diabetes Care* 2016; 39:1356–1363

Clausen TD, Mathiesen ER, Hansen T, Pedersen O, Jensen DM, Lauenborg J, Schmidt L, Damm P. Overweight and the metabolic syndrome in adult offspring of women with diet-treated gestational diabetes or type 1 diabetes. *J Clin Endocrinol Metab* 2009;94:2464–2470

Cooper MS. Disorders of calcium metabolism and parathyroid disease. *Best Pract Res Clin Endocrinol Metab* 2011;25:975–983

Cordero L, Treuer SH, Landon MB, Gabbe SG. Management of infants of diabetic mothers. *Arch Pediatr Adolesc Med* 1998;152:249–254

Cowett RM. The infant of the diabetic mother. In *Medical and Surgical Complications of Pregnancy: Effects on the Fetus and Newborn*. Sweet AY, Brown E, Eds. Chicago, IL, Year Book, 1991a, p. 302–319

Cowett RM. Neonatal glucose metabolism. In *Principles of Perinatal-Neonatal Metabolism*. Cowett RM, Ed. New York, NY, Springer-Verlag, 1991b, p. 356–389

Cowett RM. Decreased response to catecholamines in the newborn: effect on glucose kinetics in the lamb. *Metabolism* 1988a;37:736–740

Cowett RM. The metabolic sequelae in the infant of the diabetic mother. In *Endocrinology and Metabolism*. Cohen MP, Foa PP, Eds. *Controversies in Diabetes and Pregnancy*. Jovanovic L, sect. ed. New York, NY, Springer-Verlag, 1988b, p. 149–171

Cruikshank DP, Pitkin RM, Varner MW, Williams GA, Hargis GK. Calcium metabolism in diabetic mother, fetus, and newborn infant. *Am J Obstet Gynecol* 1983;145:1010–1016

Dabelea D, Hanson RL, Lindsay RS, Pettitt DJ, Imperatore G, Gabir MM, Roumain J, Bennett PH, Knowler WC. Intrauterine exposure to diabetes conveys risks for type 2 diabetes and obesity: a study of discordant sibships. *Diabetes* 2000;49:2208–2211

Dahlquist G, Kallen B. School marks for Swedish children whose mothers had diabetes during pregnancy: a population-based study. *Diabetologia* 2007;50: 1826–1831

Filan PM, Inder TE, Cameron FJ, Kean MJ, Hunt RW. Neonatal hypoglycemia and occipital cerebral injury. *J Pediatrics* 2006;148:552–555

Freinkel N, Ogata E, Metzger BE. The offspring of the mother with diabetes. In *Ellenberg and Rifkin's Diabetes Mellitus: Theory and Practice*. 4th ed. Rifkin H, Porte D Jr., Eds. New York, NY, Elsevier, 1990, p. 651

Fuhrmann K, Reiher H, Semmler K, Fischer M, Glockner E. Prevention of congenital malformations in infants of insulin dependent diabetic mothers. *Diabetes Care* 1983;6:219–223

Goldman JA, Dicker D, Feldberg D, Yeshaya A, Samuel N, Karp M. Pregnancy outcome in patients with insulin-dependent diabetes mellitus with preconceptional diabetic control: a comparative study. *Am J Obstet Gynecol* 1986;155: 193–197

Gutaj P, Wender-Ozegowska E. Diagnosis and management of IUGR in pregnancy complicated by type 1 diabetes mellitus. *Curr Diab Rep* 2016;16(5):39

Halliday HL. Hypertrophic cardiomyopathy in infants of poorly controlled diabetic mothers. *Arch Dis Child* 1981;56:258–263

Hanson U, Persson B, Stangenberg M. Factors influencing neonatal morbidity in diabetic pregnancy. *Diabetes Res Clin Pract* 1986;3:71–76

Hay WW. Care of the infant of the diabetic mother. *Curr Diab Rep* 2012;12: 4–15

Hornberger LK. Maternal diabetes and the fetal heart. *Heart* 2006;92:1019–1021

Karimzadeh P, Tabarestani S, Ghofrani M. Hypoglycemia-occipital syndrome: a specific neurologic syndrome following neonatal hypoglycemia? *J Child Neurol* 2011;26:152–159

Kitzmiller JL, Cloherty JP, Younger MD, Tabatabaii A, Rothchild SB, Sosnko I, Epstein F, Singh S, Neff RK. Diabetic pregnancy and perinatal morbidity. *Am J Obstet Gynecol* 1978;131:560–568

Koivisto M, Blanco-Sequeriros M, Krause U. Neonatal symptomatic and asymptomatic hypoglycemia; a follow-up study of 151 children. *Dev Med Child Neurol* 1972;14:603–614

Lilien LD, Pidles RS, Sainivasan G, Voora S, Yeh TF. Treatment of neonatal hypoglycemia with minibolus and intravenous glucose infusion. *J Pediatr* 1980;97:295–298

Lin HC, Maguire CA, Oh W, Cowett RM. Accuracy and reliability of glucose reflectance meters in the high-risk neonate. *J Pediatr* 1989;115:998–1000

Logan KM, Gale C, Hyde MJ, Santhakumaran S, Modi N. Diabetes in pregnancy and infant adiposity: systematic review and meta-analysis. *Arch Dis Child Fetal Neonatal Ed* 2017;102:F65–F72

Lucas A, Morley R, Cole TJ. Adverse neurodevelopmental outcome of moderate neonatal hypoglycemia. *BMJ* 1988;297:1304–1308

Mace S, Hirschfeld SS, Riggs T, Fanaroff AA, Merkatz IR. Echocardiographic abnormalities in infants of diabetic mothers. *J Pediatr* 1979;95:1013–1019

Metzger BE, Buchanan TA, Eds. Diabetes and birth defects: insights from the 1980s, prevention in the 1990s. *Diabetes Spectrum* 1990;3:149–184

Miller E, Hare JW, Cloherty JP, Dunn PJ, Gleason RE, Soeldner JS, Kitzmiller JL. Elevated maternal hemoglobin A1c in early pregnancy and major congenital anomalies in infants of diabetic mothers. *N Engl J Med* 1981;304: 1331–1334

Noguchi A, Erin M, Tsang RC. Parathyroid hormone in hypocalcemia and normocalcemic infants of diabetic mothers. *J Pediatr* 1980;97:112–114

Peevy KJ, Landaw SA, Gross SA. Hyperbilirubinemia in infants of diabetic mothers. *Pediatrics* 1980;66:417–419

Pettitt DJ, Nelson RG, Saad MF, Bennett PH, Knowler WC. Diabetes and obesity in the offspring of Pima Indian women with diabetes during pregnancy. *Diabetes Care* 1993;16:310–314

Pham MT, Brubaker K, Pruett K, Caughey AB. Risk of childhood obesity in the toddler offspring of mothers with gestational diabetes. *Obstet Gynecol* 2013;121:976–982

Philipps LH, Santhakumaran S, Gale C, Prior E, Logan KM, Hyde MJ, Modi N. The diabetic pregnancy and offspring BMI in childhood: a systematic review and meta-analysis. *Diabetologia* 2011;54:1957–1966

Reller MD, Kaplan S. Hypertrophic cardiomyopathy in infants of diabetic mothers: an update. *Am J Perinatol* 1988;4:353–358

Salvesen DR, Brudenell MJ, Nicolaides KH. Fetal polycythemia and thrombocytopenia in pregnancies complicated by maternal diabetes mellitus. *Am J Obstet Gynecol* 1992;166:1287–1292

Schwartz R, Teramo KA. Effects of diabetic pregnancy on the fetus and newborn. *Semin Perinatol* 2000;24:120–135

Sheffield JS, Butler-Koster EL, Casey BM, McIntire DD, Leveno KJ. Maternal diabetes mellitus and infant malformations. *Obstet Gynecol* 2002;100 (5 Pt. 1):925–930

Srinivasan G, Pildes RS, Cattamanchi G, Vooru S, Lilien LD. Plasma glucose values in normal neonates: a new look. *J Pediatr* 1986;109:114–117

Stenhouse E, Wright DE, Hattersley AT, Millward BA. Maternal glucose levels influence birthweight and "catch-up" and "catch-down" growth in a large contemporary cohort. *Diabet Med* 2006;234:1207–1212

Stevenson DK, Ostrander CR, Cohen RS, Johnson JD, Schwartz HC. Pulmonary excretion of carbon monoxide in the human infant as an index of bilirubin production. *Eur J Pediatr* 1981a;137:255–259

Stevenson DK, Ostrander CR, Hopper AO, Cohen RS, Johnson JD. Pulmonary excretion of carbon monoxide as an index of bilirubin production. IIa. Evidence for possible delayed clearance of bilirubin in infants of diabetic mothers. *J Pediatr* 1981b;98:822–824

Taylor PM, Wolfson J, Bright NH, Britchard EL, Derinoz MN, Watson DW. Hyperbilirubinemia in infants of diabetic mothers. *Biol Neonate* 1963;5: 289–298

Touger L, Looker HC, Krakoff J, Lindsay RS, Cook V, Knowler WC. Early growth in offspring of diabetic mothers. *Diabetes Care* 2005;28:585–589

Way GL, Wolfe RR, Eshaghpour E, Bender RL, Jaffe RB, Ruttenberg HD. The natural history of hypertrophic cardiomyopathy in infants of diabetic mothers. *J Pediatr* 1979;95:1020–1025

Wren C, Birrell G, Hawthorne G. Cardiovascular malformations in infants of diabetic mothers. *Heart* 2003;89:1217–1220

Wyatt JW, Frias JL, Hoyme HE, Jovanovic L, Kaaja R, Brown F, Garg S, Lee-Parritz A, Seely EW, Kerr L, Mattoo V, Tan M, the IONS Study Group. Congenital anomaly rate in offspring of pre-gestational diabetic women treated with insulin lispro during pregnancy. *Diabet Med* 2004;21:2001–2007

Yang J, Cummings EA, O'Connell C, Jangaard K. Fetal and neonatal outcomes of diabetic pregnancies. *Obstet Gynecol* 2006;108:644–650

Postpartum Concerns for Women with Diabetes

Highlights
Postpartum Concerns for Women with Diabetes

■ After delivery, women with preexisting diabetes can be restarted on their prepregnancy diabetes medications, although lower doses may be needed to avoid hypoglycemia.

■ For women with gestational diabetes mellitus, their diabetes medications can be discontinued after delivery, but glucose testing is needed at 4–12 weeks postpartum to determine whether they have developed prediabetes or diabetes.

■ Breast-feeding is recommended for all women with diabetes in pregnancy and has health benefits for both mother and infant.

■ All postpartum women should be encouraged to return to their prepregnancy weight by 6–12 months postpartum.

Postpartum Concerns for Women with Diabetes

The care of the postpartum patient can be divided into immediate management after delivery of the infant and the placenta through hospital discharge, and the following 12 weeks as the physiology returns to that of the prepregnancy state. The goals and challenges facing the patient and her team change over time. Counseling and preparing women for the days, weeks, and months after delivery during the antepartum period will provide her with the tools to successfully transition to motherhood.

POSTPARTUM CARE

Ideally, the patients with diabetes will have achieved excellent glycemic control approaching delivery, providing the infant with the best intrauterine environment to transition from after delivery. Infants born to women with diabetes, however, are at risk for hypoglycemia and electrolyte disturbances after delivery as the intrauterine delivery of glucose is abruptly stopped. Hospitals may have individualized protocols to identify and intervene for the hypoglycemic infant, often including formula supplementation. One intervention that allows for the mother to exclusively provide breast milk to this at-risk infant is to encourage and instruct the collection of colostrum in the late preterm and term antenatal period, for administration via syringe or spoon to the hypoglycemic infant as breast-feeding is initiated. Although early small studies suggested a risk of preterm delivery with this practice, a multicenter, unblinded, randomized controlled trial concluded there was no harm with initiating colostrum collection at 36 weeks (Forster et al. 2017).

Upon delivery, women with diabetes should have the opportunity and be encouraged to participate in skin-to-skin or kangaroo care to facilitate the infant's transition to extrauterine life, as well as promote breast-feeding. Although they have more difficulty in the beginning and have a higher fallout rate, nursing mothers with diabetes who make it past the early weeks have the same duration of breast-feeding as nursing mothers without diabetes (Ferris et al. 1993).

Women with gestational diabetes mellitus (GDM) may discontinue oral or insulin regimens immediately after the neonate delivers. Women with type 2 diabetes (T2D) may return to prepregnancy oral antidiabetic medications or continue on insulin therapy. Women with type 1 diabetes (T1D) can also return to their prepregnancy insulin regimen, although often they experience a "honeymoon" period during which they may require significantly less insulin 1–2 weeks postpartum than they did before pregnancy. We often start women with T1D on 80% of their prepregnancy insulin dose immediately after delivery. Remember that women who had cesarean deliveries may not have significant oral intake for 6–48 h, and their short-acting, meal-based insulin should be held during that time. Insulin therapy in the days following delivery is a balancing act because avoiding hypoglycemia must be a priority so that the mother can care for her infant, but glucose control is also imperative for wound healing. For women with T1D and T2D continuing self-monitoring of blood glucose (SMBG) and following the principles of the pregnancy meal plan are vital.

Typical postpartum admissions in the U.S. are <48 h for patients who deliver vaginally, and 72–96 h for women undergoing cesarean delivery. As a result, many postpartum obstetric complications become apparent after the patient has been discharged home. Because women with GDM or preexisting diabetes are at increased risk for preeclampsia and cesarean delivery (Yogev et al. 2004, Ehrenberg et al. 2004, Piccoli et al. 2013), the physician must be thorough in reviewing the signs and symptoms of postpartum preeclampsia, cardiomyopathy, and wound complications so that the patient may return for timely evaluation. Comorbidities, including vascular, renal, or retinal disease, also should be considered when evaluating individualized postpartum risks and timing for outpatient follow-up. Most low-risk patients are scheduled for a single postpartum visit around 6 weeks postpartum, but consideration should be given for a shorter interval and more frequent visits in women with diabetes to assess blood pressure and glucose control, postpartum depression screening, and lactation support.

Upon hospital discharge, women with T1D and T2D should follow up closely with the physician who manages their diabetes. If their care was inconsistent, then the importance of routine care should be stressed and an appointment made. For women with GDM, a 75-g, 2-h oral glucose tolerance test should be scheduled at 4–12 weeks postpartum to identify women who have already developed T2D or prediabetes (American Diabetes Association 2018). In the majority of cases, this test is not performed, so its importance should be stressed both before delivery and postpartum (Werner et al. 2016). Women with GDM have up to a 70% chance of developing T2D as they age. Therefore, even if women have no sign of diabetes when tested 4–12 weeks postpartum, they should be retested every 1–3 years. At any point if prediabetes is identified, lifestyle modification or metformin should be recommended. When women who have prediabetes, and also had previous GDM, were randomized to metformin treatment, lifestyle intervention, or placebo, the annual incidence of conversion to diabetes was 15% in the placebo group, but it was cut in half by treatment with either lifestyle modification or metformin (Ratner et al. 2008). Five women are needed to treat with lifestyle intervention to prevent one case of diabetes over 3 years. With the appropriate guidance to achieve weight loss and fitness goals, these women can improve their health and lower their risk of developing diabetes.

Postpartum women with diabetes are also at increased risk for postpartum thyroiditis. Although the exact cause is unknown, the etiology is thought to be autoimmune. As many as 10% of postpartum women may develop thyroiditis. Clinical course and manifestation vary but many women experience a 1- to 4-month period of hyperthyroidism in which anxiety, insomnia, palpitations, fatigue, weight loss, and irritability are common. This is followed by hypothyroidism in which women experience fatigue, weight gain, constipation, dry skin, depression, and poor exercise tolerance. This phase usually resolves by 1 year postpartum; rarely, however, women remain hypothyroid.

BREAST-FEEDING

Exclusive breast-feeding is recommended for the first 6 months of life and should continue, with supplemental calories, from 6–12 months of age, and longer as it is mutually desired by both mother and child (American Academy of Pediatrics, Section on Breastfeeding 2012, American Dietetic Association [now Academy of Nutrition and Dietetics] 2009, American College of Obstetricians and Gynecologists [ACOG] 2016). Unicef and the World Health Organization (2018) recommend breast-feeding until at least age 2 years old. The benefits of breast-feeding for women with diabetes and their infants are well established. Breast-feeding has been associated with a reduction in risk for development of T2D in women with previous GDM and in the children born to women with diabetes (Martens et al. 2016).

A review of the current evidence on the associations of breast-feeding suggests that short duration or lack of breast-feeding may be a risk factor for the development of T1D (Patelarou et al. 2012, Martens et al. 2016, Lund-Blix et al. 2017). Children of women with diabetes (preexisting and GDM), who were breast-fed for ≥6 months had reduced adiposity compared with those who were not adequately breast-fed (Crume et al. 2011). A short duration of breast-feeding (i.e., ≤4 months) and large birth weight are predictive factors for obesity in children of men and women with T1D (Hummel et al. 2009). The benefits of breast-feeding are magnified by early initiation, duration, and exclusivity.

The majority of women whose diabetes is well controlled can successfully breast-feed, but these women are at increased risk for lactation complications compared to women without diabetes (Lawrence and Lawrence 2015). Poor metabolic control during pregnancy can negatively affect serum prolactin as well as placental lactogen and mammary development, which ultimately can affect milk production (Neubauer 1990). Predictive factors for the initiation and maintenance of breast-feeding in women with T1D include establishing early breast-feeding (Sparud-Lundin et al. 2011). In addition, fluctuations in blood glucose levels after birth can impair lactose synthesis (Arthur et al. 1994, Hartmann and Cregan 2001, Oliveira et al. 2008) and delay the onset of lactogenesis an average of 15–28 h; thus, glucose control soon after birth can help to ensure breast-feeding success (Arthur et al. 1989).

Women with diabetes are also more prone to mastitis and candidal infections of the nipple and breast during lactation (Arthur et al. 1994). Optimal management of diabetes reduces such complications, and with good metabolic control, nursing mothers who have diabetes breast-feed as well as their counterparts without diabetes once they have successfully navigated any early postpartum issues (Ferris et al. 1993, Stage et al. 2006, American Dietetic Association [now Academy of Nutrition and Dietetics] 2009).

In general, lactation does not lead to significant changes in blood glucose (American Academy of Pediatrics, Section on Breastfeeding 2012). Blood glucose, however, may be more variable during lactation for women with T1D, and both hyper- and hypoglycemia are possible. The extent of variability may depend on the amount of milk produced and the frequency of feeding (Bentley-Lewis et al. 2007). Hypoglycemia is most likely to occur within 1 h after breast-feeding, so periodic SMBG at this time is encouraged to determine the need for, and timing of, snacks. Episodes of hypoglycemia may be avoided by eating a snack with at least 15 g of carbohydrate and protein (Bradley 2007). The inclusion of a snack containing carbohydrate and protein before bedtime may avoid nighttime hypoglycemia (2:00–6:00 A.M.). Adjustments to evening insulin doses also can be made. Because most women experience fatigue postpartum and sleep more frequently, albeit for shorter intervals, it is important to consider nap times that do not interfere with mealtimes to avoid hypoglycemia from missed meals. To avoid this, women should be encouraged to nap after meals and snacks, not before. Continuation of the pregnancy meal plan often is suggested, along with SMBG, to meet the glycemic targets and ensure adequate nutrition.

NUTRITION RECOMMENDATIONS

POSTPARTUM NUTRITION MANAGEMENT

The goals of medical nutrition therapy (MNT) for postpartum women with diabetes are to provide excellent nutrition for the infant being breast-fed, promote maternal blood glucose target range, and contribute to the long-term risk reduction for coronary vascular disease (Patelarou et al. 2012). Among mothers exclusively breast-feeding their infants, the energy demands of lactation exceed prepregnancy demands by ~500 kcal/day for milk production of 780 mL/day for the first 6 months of lactation (Kitzmiller et al. 2008) (Table 8.1). Postpartum calorie needs for women are a minimum of 1,800 kcal/day. Individual energy needs vary depending on breast-feeding status and production volume, the amount of stored maternal fat, and the woman's energy expenditure (Reader and Franz 2004). Table 8.2 includes the dietary reference intakes (DRI) for breast-feeding women. These women need to meet their own postpartum nutritional needs as well as produce an adequate volume of milk to meet their babies' nutritional needs.

Table 8.1—Energy Adjustments for Lactation

Lactation	EER = prepregnancy EER + milk energy output – weight loss since delivery
First 6 months	EER + 500 – 170 kcal/day
Second 6 months	EER + 400 kcal/day – 0

EER, estimated energy requirements.

Source: Adapted from Institute of Medicine, Food and Nutrition Board (2006).

Table 8.2—Dietary Reference Intakes for Women[a]

Nutrient	Adult Woman	Pregnancy	Lactation (0–6 months)
Energy (kcal)	2,403	2,743[b], 2,855[c]	2,698
Protein (g/kg/d)	0.8	1.1	1.1
Carbohydrate (g/d)	130	175	210
Total fiber (g/d)	25	28	29
Fluids, l/day (cups/d)	2.2 (~9)	2.3 (~10)	3.1 (~13)
Linoleic acid (g/d)	12	13	13
α-Linolenic acid (g/d)	12	13	13
Vitamin A (µg RAE)[d]	700	770	1,300
Vitamin D (µg)[e,f]	10	10	10
Vitamin E (mg α-tocopherol)	15	15	19
Vitamin K (µg)	90	90	90
Vitamin C (mg)	75	85	120
Thiamin (mg)	1.1	1.4	1.4
Riboflavin (mg)	1.1	1.4	1.6
Vitamin B_6 (mg)	1.3	1.9	2.0
Niacin (mg NE)[g]	14	18	17
Folate (µg dietary folate equivalents)	400	600	500
Vitamin B_{12} (µg)	2.4	2.6	2.8
Pantothenic acid (mg)	5	6	7
Biotin (µg)	30	30	35
Choline (mg)	425	450	550
Calcium (mg)	1,000	1,000	1,000
Phosphorus (mg)	700	700	700
Magnesium (mg)	320	350	310
Iron (mg)	18	27	19
Zinc (mg)	8	11	12
Iodine (µg)	150	220	290
Selenium (µg)	55	60	70
Fluoride (mg)	3	3	3
Manganese (mg)	1.8	2.0	2.6

(continues p. 132)

Table 8.2 (continued)

Nutrient	Adult Woman	Pregnancy	Lactation (0–6 months)
Molybdenum (µg)	45	50	50
Chromium (µg)	25	30	45
Copper (µg)	900	1,000	1,300
Sodium (mg)	2,300	2,300	2,300
Potassium (mg)	4,700	4,700	5,100

[a] Values are recommended dietary allowances except energy (estimated energy requirement) and total fiber, linoleic acid, α-linolenic acid, vitamin K, pantothenic acid, biotin, choline, manganese, chromium, sodium, and potassium (adequate intakes).

[b] Second trimester for women ages 19–50 years.

[c] Third trimester for women ages 19–50 years.

[d] RAE = retinol activity equivalents.

[e] As cholecalciferol: 1 µg cholecalciferol = 40 IU vitamin D.

[f] Under the assumption of minimal sunlight.

[g] NE = niacin equivalents: 1 mg niacin = 60 mg tryptophan.

Source: Data from Institute of Medicine, Food and Nutrition Board (2006, 2010).

Returning to prepregnancy weight by 6–12 months postpartum is an important goal for all postpartum women. Increased emphasis and support should be provided for women with diabetes who are overweight (body mass index [BMI] 25–30 kg/m²) or obese (BMI ≥30 kg/m²) to reduce their weight to a BMI ≤25 kg/m² (Nicklas and Barbour 2015). Moderate weight loss and cardiovascular disease risk reduction may be achieved by balancing caloric intake and physical activity (150 min/week) (American Diabetes Association 2008). Referral to a registered dietitian nutritionist can be especially helpful. Nutrition recommendations for managing diabetes in women may be implemented (American Diabetes Association 2018). Women should be encouraged to continue healthy eating changes made during pregnancy to benefit lifelong health.

The relationship between breast-feeding and weight loss is neither consistent nor conclusive. Women who are breast-feeding should be given realistic, health-promoting advice about weight changes during lactation. Many women lose weight during the first 6 months of lactation, but some women maintain weight. The average rate of weight loss is ~0.5–1 kg/month (~1–2 lb/month) after the first month postpartum, with 1–2 kg/month (4–5 lb) acceptable for women who are overweight (Lovelady et al. 2000). Rapid weight loss (>2 kg/month [>4.4 lb/month] after the first month postpartum) is not advised for breast-feeding women. Intakes of <1,500 kcal/day have resulted in decreased milk output (Strode et al. 1986). Extreme diets and weight-loss medications are not recommended. A registered dietitian nutritionist can assist women who wish to lose weight safely.

MACRONUTRIENTS

To meet the additional demand during lactation, the estimated average requirement (EAR) for carbohydrates is 160 g/day with a recommended daily allowance (RDA) of 210 g/day (Institute of Medicine [IOM] 2006). This should be sufficient carbohydrate for an adequate volume of milk, to prevent ketonemia, and to maintain appropriate glucose levels during lactation (Reader and Franz 2004). Diets with little or no carbohydrates are not safe in pregnancy or when lactating and should be avoided. Fat intake approximates 20–35% of energy. The adequate intake for essential fatty acids is the same as during pregnancy, 13 g/day of omega-6 (n-6) fatty acids and 1.4 g/day of omega-3 (n-3) fatty acids (IOM 2009). Inclusion of 8–12 oz of seafood per week is recommended, given the mercury concerns for pregnancy reviewed in Chapter 3 (American Diabetes Association 2018). The RDA for protein in lactation is set to preserve muscle and maintain milk production. The EAR for protein is 1.05 g/kg/day with an RDA of 71 g/day (IOM 2006, Reader and Franz 2004). Breast-feeding mothers do not need to drink large amounts of fluids to produce sufficient milk; they should be advised to drink to thirst. Total water intake includes drinking water and other beverages, but also fluids as part of foods (~22%) (Kitzmiller et al. 2008). The DRI for water in lactation is 13 cups/day or 9–10 cups of beverages. Encouraging mothers to sip on a beverage (preferably water or caffeine-free tea) while nursing, with a goal of keeping their urine a pale yellow color, may be a helpful guideline.

MICRONUTRIENTS

Women with preexisting diabetes should be encouraged to continue with a nutrient-dense diet (see Chapter 3). During the postpartum period, the need for supplementation depends on the woman's nutritional status. A prenatal vitamin is recommended in women who are lactating. Women found to be anemic after delivery or at their postpartum checkup are encouraged to take 60–120 mg/day of elemental iron daily until the anemia is resolved (ACOG 2008). Women at higher risk for nutritional deficiencies, such as women with a history of gastric bypass surgery, may require a multivitamin–mineral supplement. Vegetarian women also may need supplementation of vitamin B_{12} (IOM 2006).

SELECTED READINGS

Academy of Nutrition and Dietetics (formerly American Dietetic Association). *Medical Nutrition Therapy, Evidence-Based Guides for Practice: Gestational Diabetes Mellitus Evidence-Based Guide for Practice.* Chicago, American Dietetic Association, 2008

Academy of Nutrition and Dietetics (formerly American Dietetic Association). *Medical Nutrition Therapy, Evidence-Based Guides for Practice: Type 1 & 2 Diabetes Mellitus Evidence-Based Guide for Practice.* Chicago, American Dietetic Association, 2008

American Diabetes Association. Management of diabetes in pregnancy: standards of medical care in diabetes, 2018. *Diabetes Care* 2018;41(Suppl. 1):S137–S143

Thomas A. Pregnancy with pre-existing diabetes. In *The Art and Science of Diabetes Self-Management Education. A Desk Reference for Healthcare Professionals.* Messing C, Ed. Chicago, IL, American Association of Diabetes Educators, 2006

REFERENCES

American Academy of Pediatrics, Section on Breastfeeding. Breastfeeding and the use of human milk. *Pediatrics* 2012;129(3):e827–e841. PMID: 22371471

American College of Obstetricians and Gynecologists. Practice bulletin no. 95: Anemia in pregnancy. *Obstet Gynecol* 2008;112:201–207. PMID: 18591330

American College of Obstetricians and Gynecologists' Committee on Obstetric Practice; Breastfeeding Expert Work Group. Committee opinion no. 658: Optimizing support for breastfeeding as part of obstetric practice. *Obstet Gynecol* 2016;127(2):e86–e92. PMID: 26942393

American Diabetes Association. Managing preexisting diabetes for pregnancy. Consensus statement. *Diabetes Care* 2008;31:1060–1079. PMID: 18445730

American Diabetes Association. Management of diabetes in pregnancy: standards of medical care in diabetes, 2018. *Diabetes Care* 2018;41(Suppl. 1):S137–S143. PMID: 29222384

American Dietetic Association (now Academy of Nutrition and Dietetics). Position of the American Dietetic Association: promoting and supporting breastfeeding. *J Am Diet Assoc* 2009;109:1926–1942. PMID: 19862847

Arthur PG, Kent JC, Hartmann PE. Metabolites of lactose synthesis in milk from diabetic and nondiabetic women during lactogenesis II. *J Pediatr Gastroenterol Nutr* 1994;19:100–108. PMID: 7965458

Arthur PG, Smith M, Hartmann PE. Milk lactose, citrate, and glucose as markers of lactogenesis in normal and diabetic women. *J Pediatr Gastroenterol Nutr* 1989;9:488–496. PMID: 2621526

Bentley-Lewis R, Goldfine AB, Green DE, Seely EW. Lactation after normal pregnancy is not associated with blood glucose fluctuations. *Diabetes Care* 2007;30:2792–2793. PMID: 17698611

Bradley C. Managing diabetes while breast-feeding. *Diabetes Self Manag* 2007;24(2):84, 87–89. PMID: 17410675

Crume TL, Ogden L, Maligie MB, Sheffield S, Bischoff K, McDuffie R, Daniels S, Hamman RF, Norris JM, Dabelea D. Long-term impact of neonatal breast-feeding on childhood adiposity and fat distribution among children exposed to diabetes in utero. *Diabetes Care* 2011;34:641–645. PMID: 21357361

Ehrenberg HM, Durnwald CP, Catalano P, Mercer BM. The influence of obesity and diabetes on the risk of cesarean delivery. *Am J Obstet Gynecol* 2004;191: 969–974. PMID: 15467574

Ferris AM, Neubauer SH, Bendel RB, Green KW, Ingardia CJ, Reece EA. Perinatal lactation protocol and outcome in mothers with and without insulin-dependent diabetes mellitus. *Am J Clin Nutr* 1993;58:43–48. PMID: 8317388

Forster DA, Moorhead AM, Jacobs SE, Davis PG, Walker SP, McEgan KM, Opie GF, Donath SM, Gold L, McNamara C, Aylward A, East C, Ford R, Amir LH. Advising women with diabetes in pregnancy to express breastmilk in late pregnancy (Diabetes and Antenatal Milk Expressing [DAME]): a multicentre, unblinded, randomised controlled trial. *Lancet* 2017;389(10085): 2204–2213. PMID: 28589894

Hartmann P, Cregan M. Lactogenesis and the effects of insulin-dependent diabetes mellitus and prematurity. *J Nutr* 2001;131:3016S–3020S. PMID: 16317163

Hummel S, Pfluger M, Kriechauf S, Hummel M, Ziegler AG. Predictors of overweight during childhood in offspring of parents with type 1 diabetes. *Diabetes Care* 2009;32:921–925. PMID: 19228867

Institute of Medicine, Food and Nutrition Board. *Dietary Reference Intakes: The Essential Guide to Nutrient Requirements.* Washington, DC, The National Academies Press, 2006

Institute of Medicine, Food and Nutrition Board. *Dietary Reference Intakes for Calcium and Vitamin D.* Washington, DC, The National Academies Press, 2010

Institute of Medicine, National Research Council. *Weight Gain During Pregnancy: Reexamining the Guidelines.* Rasmussen KM, Taktine AL, Eds. Washington, DC, The National Academies Press, 2009

Kitzmiller JL, Jovanovic L, Brown FM, Coustan DR, Reader DM (Eds.). *Managing Preexisting Diabetes and Pregnancy: Technical Reviews and Consensus Recommendations for Care.* Alexandria, VA, American Diabetes Association, 2008

Lawrence RA, Lawrence RM. *Breastfeeding: A Guide for the Medical Profession.* 8th ed. Philadelphia, PA, Elsevier Mosby, 2015

Lovelady CA, Garner KE, Moreno KL, Williams JP. The effect of weight loss in overweight, lactating women on the growth of their infants. *N Engl J Med* 2000;342:449–453. PMID: 10675424

Lund-Blix NA, Dydensborg Sander S, Størdal K, Nybo Andersen AM, Rønningen KS, Joner G, Skrivarhaug T, Njølstad PR, Husby S, Stene LC. Infant feeding and risk of type 1 diabetes in two large Scandinavian birth cohorts. *Diabetes Care* 2017;40(7):920–927. PMID: 28487451

Martens PJ, Shafer LA, Dean HJ, Sellers EA, Yamamoto J, Ludwig S, Heaman M, Phillips-Beck W, Prior HJ, Morris M, McGavock J, Dart AB, Shen GX. Breastfeeding initiation associated with reduced incidence of diabetes in mothers and offspring. *Obstet Gynecol* 2016;128(5):1095–1104. PMID: 27741196

Neubauer SH. Lactation in insulin-dependent diabetes. *Prog Food Nutr Sci* 1990;14:333–370. PMID: 2091054

Nicklas JM, Barbour LA. Optimizing weight for maternal and infant health – tenable, or too late? *Expert Rev Endocrinol Metab* 2015;10(2):227–242

Oliveira AM, da Cunha CC, Penha-Silva N, Abdallah VO, Jorge PT. [Interference of the blood glucose control in the transition between phases I and II of lactogenesis in patients with type 1 diabetes mellitus]. *Arq Bras Endocrinol Metabol* 2008;52:473–481. PMID: 18506272

Patelarou E, Girvalaki C, Brokalaki H, Patelarou A, Androulaki Z, Vardavas C. Current evidence on the associations of breastfeeding, infant formula, and cow's milk introduction with type 1 diabetes mellitus: a systematic review. *Nutr Rev* 2012;70:509–519. PMID: 22946851

Piccoli GB, Clari R, Ghiotto, S, Castelluccia N, Colombi N, Mauro G, Tavassoli E, Melluzza C, Cabiddu G, Gernone G, Mongilardi E, Ferraresi M, Rolfo A, Todros T. Type 1 diabetes, diabetic nephropathy, and pregnancy: a systematic review and meta-study. *Rev Diabet Stud* 2013;10(1):6–26. PMID: 24172695

Ratner RE, Christophi CA, Metzger BE, Dabelea D, Bennett P, Pi-Sunyer X, Fowler S, Kahn SE. Prevention of diabetes in women with a history of gestational diabetes: effects of metformin and lifestyle intervention. *Clin Endocrinol Metab* 2008;93:4774–4779

Reader D, Franz MJ. Lactation, diabetes and nutrition recommendations. *Curr Diabetes Rep* 2004;4:370–376. PMID: 15461903

Sparud-Lundin C, Wennergren N, Elfvin A, Berg M. Breastfeeding in women with type 1 diabetes: exploration of predictive factors. *Diabetes Care* 2011;34: 296–301. PMID: 21270187

Stage E, Norgard H, Damm P, Mathiesen E. Long-term breast-feeding in women with type 1 diabetes. *Diabetes Care* 2006;29:771–774. PMID: 16567813

Strode MA, Dewey KG, Lonnerdal B. Effects of short-term caloric restriction on lactational performance of well-nourished women. *Acta Paediatr Scand* 1986;75:222–229. PMID: 3754376

Werner EF, Has P, Tarabulsi G, Lee J, Satin A. Early postpartum glucose testing in women with gestational diabetes mellitus. *Am J Perinatol* 2016;33(10): 966–971. PMID: 27120481

World Health Organization. Infant and young children feeding fact sheet. Updated 16 February 2018. Available from www.who.int/mediacentre/factsheets/fs342/en/. Accessed 28 February 2019

Yogev Y, Xenakis EM, Langer O. The association between preeclampsia and the severity of gestational diabetes: the impact of glycemic control. *Am J Obstet Gynecol* 2004;191:1655–1660. PMID: 15547538

Contraception in Women with Diabetes and Prior Gestational Diabetes Mellitus

Highlights
Contraception in Women with Diabetes and Prior Gestational Diabetes Mellitus

■ Use of a safe and efficacious contraceptive method is integral to avoid unplanned pregnancy and achieve optimal health for women with diabetes. When counseling women, comorbid conditions, including those not associated with diabetes, must be considered as well as the woman's lifestyle, individual preferences, and ease of use of the contraceptive method.

■ Standard guidelines recommended to monitor glycemic control, serum lipid levels, blood pressure, and renal and retinal surveillance should be evaluated and considered when prescribing contraceptives in all women with diabetes or prediabetes.

■ The copper and levonorgestrel-releasing intrauterine devices (IUD) are metabolically neutral and have been shown to be highly efficacious in women with diabetes and other comorbidities. They do not increase the risk of pelvic inflammatory disease.

■ Estrogen-containing methods, including combination oral contraceptives, vaginal rings, and transdermal patches, should not be prescribed to women with diabetic sequelae (retinopathy, nephropathy, or neuropathy), hypertension or other cardiovascular disease, or increased coagulation risk, or during the first 6 weeks after delivery. These methods are not appropriate for women who have comorbidities, not related to diabetes, that are contraindications to estrogen supplementation.

■ Progestin-only methods, including progestin-only oral contraceptives, injectables, subcutaneous implants, and progestin-releasing IUD, do not affect blood pressure levels or coagulation factors and have minimal lipid metabolic effects.

■ Women with prior gestational diabetes mellitus and normal postpartum glucose tolerance can use all methods of contraception.

■ Once childbearing is completed, permanent sterilization is a highly efficacious method to prevent unplanned pregnancy and can be accomplished via surgical ligation, salpingectomy, or hysteroscopic surgical tubal occlusion.

Contraception in Women with Diabetes and Prior Gestational Diabetes Mellitus

When counseling and providing contraceptives to women with diabetes or a history of gestational diabetes mellitus (GDM), the healthcare provider must consider not only the general risks and benefits of contraceptive methods but also a woman's existing comorbidities and the metabolic effects of the contraceptive methods. Equally important is the consequence of an unplanned pregnancy for the woman and her potential offspring. Should pregnancy occur when glycemic targets are not being met, the likelihood of major congenital anomalies is ~20–23% (Miller et al. 1981), and the combined risk of congenital anomalies and spontaneous abortion when glycemic targets are not being met in early pregnancy can approach 65% (Greene 1993). Effective contraception allows a woman and her physician to plan pregnancy when glycemic targets are met (hemoglobin A_{1c} [A1C] <7%), reducing the risk of anomalies. Pregnancy planning also enables a woman to optimize her health with respect to other risk factors, such as body mass index, hypertension, and microvascular disease, ultimately reducing her risks for pregnancy complications. When selecting a contraceptive method for women with diabetes or prior GDM, glycemia, serum lipid levels, blood pressure, and renal and retinal health should all be considered.

The practitioner's goal is to prescribe the contraceptive method that poses the least risk relating to her diabetes, has the greatest efficacy, and is acceptable to the woman. Therefore, each patient's acceptance of side effects, her comfort with the method, and her ability to successfully use her chosen method must all be considered. Although the method may not be risk free, individualized counseling, lifestyle interventions, and adequate management of her disease process generally can minimize these risks to an acceptable level. This chapter will deal with methods that have higher efficacy, primarily long-acting reversible contraceptives; oral, injectable, and transvaginal hormonal methods; and sterilization. Barrier methods, including spermicides, the diaphragm, condoms, cervical caps, and contraceptive sponges, will not be considered in detail as there are no medical contraindications to their use except higher failure rates (Table 9.1).

Table 9.1—Continuation Rate and Unintended Pregnancy Rate during the First Year of Typical and Perfect Use in the U.S. by Birth Control Method

Method	Continuation at 1 Year	Pregnancy Rate During: Typical Use	Perfect Use
Sterilization			
Female sterilization	100%	0.5%	0.5%
Male sterilization	100%	0.15%	0.1%
Hormonal Long-Acting Reversible Contraception (LARC)			
LNG-IUS (Mirena, Skyla, Kyleena, Liletta)	80%	0.2%	0.2%
Implant (Nexplanon)	84%	0.05%	0.05%
Nonhormonal LARC			
Copper intrauterine device (Paragard)	78%	0.8%	0.6%
Estrogen/Progestin Methods			
Combination oral contraceptives (COC)	67%	9%	0.3%
Transdermal patch (Evra)	67%	9%	0.3%
Vaginal ring (NuvaRing)	67%	9%	0.3%
Progestin-Only Methods			
Progestin-only oral contraceptive (PO-OC)	67%	9%	0.3%
DMPA injection (Depo-Provera)	56%	6%	0.2%
Barrier Methods			
Spermicides	42%	28%	18%
Vaginal sponge (parous/nulliparous)	36%	24% / 12%	20% / 9%
Diaphragm	57%	12%	6%
Male condom	43%	18%	2%
Female condom	41%	21%	5%
Low Efficacy			
No method		85%	85%
Withdrawal	46%	22%	4%
Fertility awareness (rhythm method)	47%	24%	0.4–5%

LNG-IUS, Levonorgestrel-releasing intrauterine system.

Source: Adapted from Trussell (2011).

HORMONAL CONTRACEPTIVES BACKGROUND

Reproductive-age women produce estrogen and progesterone. Hormonal contraception options are contraindicated in women in whom additional hormones may not be adequately metabolized and in women in whom hormones may accelerate their underlying disease process.

Estrogen does not provide contraception, but it does help in cycle control when given in combination with progestins. Estrogen-plus-progestin methods are most widely prescribed as combination oral contraceptives (COC), but they also are available transdermally (Evra patch) and vaginally (NuvaRing), or through monthly combination injectable contraceptives (CIC), which currently are off the market. Estrogen generally has a desirable effect on serum lipid levels (lowering low-density lipoprotein cholesterol, increasing high-density lipoprotein cholesterol) and will produce a mild increase in triglycerides. These effects are mediated largely through the first pass through the liver, after absorption from the gut. Estrogen also has no effect on insulin resistance. However, estrogen produces a dose-dependent increase in liver-produced globulins, thereby increasing coagulation factors, the risk for a thrombotic event, angiotensin II levels, and mean arterial blood pressure (Meade 1982, Godsland et al. 1990). Therefore, women with diabetes or prediabetes who have vascular sequelae, hypertension, or cardiovascular disease (or if they smoke or have prior thrombotic disease, such as factor V Leiden) should not use estrogen-containing contraceptives, and the U.S. Medical Eligibility Criteria (U.S. MEC 2010) has assigned these contraceptives a category 3/4 risk. A category 3 designation is given when theoretical or proven risks usually outweigh the advantages, and a category 4 designation is given when health risks are unacceptable (Table 9.2).

LONG-ACTING REVERSIBLE CONTRACEPTIVES: INTRAUTERINE DEVICES AND IMPLANTS

INTRAUTERINE DEVICES

The guidelines for use of intrauterine devices (IUDs) in women with diabetes follow the same guidelines as for all women—offered routinely as a first-line contraceptive to nulliparous and parous women, adolescent and adult. Among women 15–44 years old, use of IUDs increased by 83% from 2006–2010 (3.5%) to 2011–2013 (6.4%) based on the most recently available data from the National Survey of Family Growth (Branum and Jones 2015).

Table 9.2—Contraception Options for Women with Diabetes and Other Associated Conditions and Assessment of Risks Based on the U.S. Medical Eligibility Criteria for Contraceptive Use

Condition	Sub-Condition	CHC		POP		Injection		Implant		LNG-IUD		Cu-IUD	
		I	C	I	C	I	C	I	C	I	C	I	C
Age		Menarche to <40=1, >40=2		Menarche to >45=1		Menarche to <18=2, 18–45=1, >45=2		Menarche to >45=1		Menarche to <20=2, >20=1		Menarche to <20=2, >20=1	
Diabetes	a) Hx GDM only	1		1		1		1		1		1	
	b) Non-vascular Disease	2		2		2		2		2		1	
	c) Nephropathy, Retinopathy, Neuropathy	3	4	2		3		2		2		1	
	d) Other vascular disease or DM >20 years duration	3	4	2		3		2		2		1	
Hypertension	a) Adequately controlled	3		1		2		1		1		1	
	b) SBP 140–159 or DBP 90–99	3		1		2		1		1		1	
	c) SBP >160 or DBP >100	4		2		3		2		2		1	
	d) Vascular disease	4		2		3		2		2		1	
History HTN in pregnancy		2		1		1		1		1		1	
Obesity	a) >30 kg/m² BMI	2		1		1		1		1		1	
	b) Menarche to 18yo with >30 kg/m² BMI	2		1		2		1		1		1	

Table 9.2 (continued)

History							
Bariatric Surgery	a) Restrictive procedure	1	1	1	1	1	1
	b) Malabsorptive procedures	COC=3 Patch/Ring=1	3	1	1	1	1
Endometrial Hyperplasia		1	1	1	1	1	1
Postpartum	a) <10 minutes after delivery of the placenta					1	2
	b) 10 minutes to <4 weeks after delivery of placenta					2	2
	c) >4 weeks postpartum					1	1
	d) Puerperal sepsis					4	4
	e) <21 days	4	1	1	1		
	f) 21 to 42 days i) with other VTE risk factors	3	1	1	1		
	f) 21 to 42 days II) without other VTE risk factors	2	1	1	1		
	c) >42 days	1	1	1	1		
Breast-feeding	a) <1 month postpartum	3	2	2	2		
	b) >1 month postpartum	2	1	1	1		
Hyperlipidemia		2/3	2	2	2	1	2

Abbreviations: C=continuation of contraceptive method; CHC=combined hormonal contraceptive (pill, patch, and ring); COC=combined oral contraceptive; Cu-IUD=copper-containing intrauterine device; I=initiation of contraceptive method; LNG-IUD=levonorgestrel-releasing intrauterine device; POP=progestin-only pill; P/R=patch/ring.

LEGEND		
1	No restriction (method may be used)	3 Theoretical or proven risks generally outweigh the advantages
2	Advantages generally outweigh theoretical or proven risks	4 Unacceptable health risk (method not to be used)

CDC — Centers for Disease Control and Prevention. National Center for Chronic Disease Prevention and Health Promotion.

Source: Adapted from U.S. Medical Eligibility Criteria for Contraceptive Use (2010).

Four levonorgestrel (LNG)-releasing IUDs (Table 9.3) are currently marketed in the U.S., and they all have a similar mechanism of action: preventing fertilization through changes in the amount and viscosity of cervical mucous, effectively making it impenetrable to sperm.

Table 9.3—Levonogestrel-Releasing IUDs

Name	Total Dose (mg)	Daily Dose (mg)	Approved Duration (years)	Size
Mirena Bayer	52	20	5	32 mm × 32 mm
Liletta Allergan		18.6	4	32 mm × 32 mm
Kyleena Bayer	19.5	17.5	5	28 mm × 30 mm
Skyla Bayer	13.5	14	3	29 mm × 30 mm

The Mirena IUD (LNG-20) releases approximately 10% of the dose and reaches 5% of the plasma level of a 105-mcg dose of oral LNG. Thus, its systemic metabolic effect appears to be minimal, but it does exert a local progestin effect on the endometrium, decreasing menstrual blood loss. It is an excellent choice for women with diabetes or a history of GDM who have heavy menses or who are at risk for endometrial hyperplasia (e.g., obese, oligomenorrhea, or polycystic ovarian syndrome). In a study of women with existing complex atypical hyperplasia or early-grade endometrial cancer, use of LNG-IUD therapy resulted in return to normal histology for the majority of patients (Pal et al. 2018). The other commercially available LNG-IUDs offer different hormonal doses and sizes that allow the patient and her physician to choose an IUD that is most suited to her needs and goals.

The copper IUD (Cu-IUD) is an excellent, nonhormonal choice. Contraception is achieved through prevention of fertilization by inhibiting sperm migration and decreased sperm viability. It is metabolically neutral and offers pregnancy protection for 10 years. One drawback is increased menstrual blood loss, which can be counteracted by daily iron supplementation or multivitamins and minerals.

Historically, the early introduction of IUDs in the U.S. was fraught with concerns about pelvic inflammatory disease (PID). Given that women with diabetes were uniquely poised to have higher complications from any infectious processes, including PID, rigorous investigation was performed to evaluate whether women with diabetes were candidates for this long-acting reversible contraceptive method. In a large meta-analysis of several prospective World Health Organization (WHO) trials, the overall incidence of PID associated with Cu-IUD use was 1.6 per 1,000 women-years of IUD use (U.S. MEC 2010). A 2013 systematic review concluded that both Cu-IUDs and LNG-IUDs are safe and effective for people with type 1 diabetes (T1D) and type 2 diabetes (T2D); no metabolic changes were identified in women with T1D, although women with T2D have not been adequately studied to make the same claim (Goldstuck and Steyn 2013).

The risk categories for hormonal and Cu-IUDs in women with T1D, T2D, and GDM are highlighted in Table 9.2. The Cu-IUD is given a risk category of 1 for women with all types of diabetes; the LNG-IUD is given a risk category of 1 for women with a history of GDM and a risk category of 2 for women with T1D and T2D (U.S. MEC 2010).

IMPLANTS

As of 2012, Nexplanon (Merck) was the only hormonal contraceptive implant in the U.S. It contains 68 mg of etonogestrel surrounded by ethylene vinyl acetate copolymer skin and is placed subdermally to allow for controlled release of etonogestrel over 3 years. The implant is 4 cm in length and 2 mm in diameter, and it is preloaded in a disposable sterile applicator. Nexplanon is an improved design from the original Implanon marketed in the U.S. in 2006; the newer version is opaque and easily identified on X-ray.

The primary mechanism of action of the implant is to suppress ovulation, although additional contraceptive means may be accomplished by thickening of the cervical mucous and alterations in the endometrial lining. One small study showed no significant metabolic changes on glucose, lipids, albuminuria, or retinal vasculature over 2 years in insulin-treated women using the etonogestrel implant (Vicente et al. 2008). The implant carries a risk category of 1 for women with a history of GDM and risk category of 2 for women with T1D and T2D (U.S. MEC 2010).

NON-LARC HORMONAL CONTRACEPTIVES

COMBINED ESTROGEN AND PROGESTIN CONTRACEPTIVES

Women with prior GDM or diabetes without vascular disease or hypertension are candidates for combination methods, including COC, transdermal patch, or vaginal ring. The U.S. MEC has assigned COC use a category 2 risk in women with diabetes who do not have vascular disease and a category 1 risk in women with prior GDM based on studies showing no increase in risk of developing diabetes with COC use (Table 9.2). Studies also have shown no increased risk in the development of diabetes with low-dose COC use in women with prior GDM (Skouby et al. 1985, 1987; Kjos et al. 1990, 1998; Kim et al. 2002).

Currently, it is not clear whether transdermal patches, vaginal rings, or monthly injections offer a metabolic advantage over COC. Small studies examining the vaginal ring in women without diabetes and in women with T1D have found no difference in glucose metabolism, lipid levels, or hemostasis compared to women using COC (Grigoryan et al. 2008). Thus, the route of combination contraceptives should be based on patient preference, expected reliability in administration of method (daily, weekly, or monthly), and reversibility (greater delay in return of fertility with CIC, currently off the market).

When selecting a COC, the formulations with the lowest possible dose or potency of both estrogen (20–35 mcg) and progestin should be selected as a general rule to reduce side effects. This strategy has been supported in several short-term and prospective studies in women with T1D who were followed for up to 1 year with lower doses of the older progestins, including norethindrone (≤0.75 mg mean daily dose), or triphasic levonorgestrel preparation; and the newer progestins, including gestodene or desogestrel. All formulations were found to have minimal effect on glycemia, lipid metabolism, and cardiovascular risk factors. Retrospective, cross-sectional studies and case-control trials in women with T1D have not found any increased risk of or progression of diabetic sequelae (retinopathy, renal disease, or hypertension) with past or current use of oral contraceptives.

Most progestins are testosterone derivatives and have varying degrees of androgenic effects (e.g., decreasing sex-binding globulin, increasing insulin resistance, and causing adverse changes in serum lipids). Newer formulations of oral progestins (desogestrel, gestodene, drospirenone) with decreased androgenicity or older, lower-dose and -potency norethindrone minimize androgenic side effects; therefore, these formulations generally should be selected (Speroff and DeCherney 1993). Consideration of which COC formulation to prescribe is especially important for women when hirsutism should be minimized (e.g., polycystic ovarian syndrome).

PROGESTIN-ONLY CONTRACEPTIVES

Most women who are not able to use estrogen, yet desire a hormonal method, will be candidates for progestin-only methods. Importantly, for women with hypertension, cardiovascular disease, and risk of thrombosis, progestin-only formulations do not affect liver globulin production and thereby do not increase blood pressure or coagulation factors (Meade 1982, Wilson et al. 1984).

Progestin-only methods can be delivered orally (PO-OC) or by injection, as implants, or through the uterine cavity (IUD). There are two formulations of PO-OC, one containing norethindrone (0.35 mg daily) and the other containing levonorgestrel (0.75 mg daily); both are taken daily with no placebo periods.

Alternative longer-acting routes of progestin-only contraception include injections given every 3 months (depo-medroxyprogesterone acetate, DMPA), subcutaneous implants (etonogestrel) every 3 years, and IUDs (levonorgestrel) every 3–5 years (implants and IUDs were discussed previously). Currently, minimal literature exists comparing the metabolic effects in women to distinguish among the various doses and routes of progestins. DMPA has been shown to have more adverse effects on lipids and insulin resistance compared with Norplant in several studies in women without diabetes or hyperlipidemia (Deslypere et al. 1985, Liew et al. 1985, Xiang et al. 2006, Lopez et al. 2014). Thus, DMPA is not used as a first-line progestin agent for women with cardiovascular disease risk factors, including coronary artery disease, history of stroke, diabetes with vascular disease, polycystic ovarian syndrome, and obesity (category 3). Some studies have suggested that long-term use of DMPA is associated with an increased risk of osteoporosis. Women who have stopped DMPA, however, appear to have similar bone density to women who have never taken DMPA, suggesting that any effects are short lived (Banks et al. 2001). Compared to other progesterone-only options, DMPA has a longer return of fertility after discontinuation and has been associated with weight gain. Oral progestins have the advantage of being more widely studied and have a better-documented safety profile. With oral progestins, women are able to rapidly discontinue therapy if side effects occur. This can be useful when given as trial therapy to see whether women can tolerate progestin side effects before administering a longer-acting injectable or implant progestin. Without clearly demonstrated metabolic differences, the various routes of administration can be determined by considering the woman's preferences regarding lifestyle, convenience, and reliability.

Studies of women with T1D have shown little to no metabolic effect of the norethindrone PO-OC on glucose and lipid metabolism (Lopez et al. 2014). PO-OCs often are reserved for women in whom estrogen is contraindicated or for patients who decline LARC or DMPA.

PERMANENT STERILIZATION

For the individual with diabetes who desires permanent prevention of future pregnancy, permanent surgical sterilization of either the woman or her partner offers an excellent contraceptive option. Sterilization can be done surgically by laparoscopy or mini-laparotomy with different methods conveying different risks if a subsequent pregnancy should occur. Whether surgical sterilization is performed at the time of delivery or remotely, prophylactic bilateral salpingectomy should be offered and discussed to reduce the risk of ovarian cancer (American College of Obstetricians and Gynecologists [ACOG] 2015). For the woman undergoing cesarean delivery, salpingectomy can be performed concurrently with minimal addition to surgical time and no change in morbidity (Shinar et al. 2017). Immediate postpartum sterilization also can be offered to women who deliver vaginally, although the need to continue fasting while maintaining glycemic targets and separation from her infant must be considered. Evaluation of salpingectomy performed at the time of mini-laparotomy also suggests promising results with similar rates of complications without a significant increase in operative time (Danis et al. 2016).

An alternative to surgical sterilization is Essure, in which flexible coils are inserted into the fallopian tubes via hysteroscopy, causing tubal scarring and occlusion within 3 months. A hysterosalpingogram is performed 3 months after the original procedure to document tubal occlusion. This method may be offered in an office setting, avoiding general anesthesia and surgery.

The pregnancy rate after sterilization of men is 0.015% and women is 0.5% (Table 9.4). Those pregnancies that do occur in sterilized women, however, are more likely to be ectopically implanted and therefore life threatening. Conversely, if male surgical sterilization occurs, and the marriage or relationship dissolves, the women with diabetes would remain susceptible to pregnancy.

Table 9.4—Pregnancy Rates by Sterilization Method

Method	5-Year (per 1,000 procedures)	10-Year (per 1,000 procedures)	Ectopic Pregnancy (per 1,000 procedures)
Postpartum partial salpingectomy	6.3	7.5	1.5
Bipolar coagulation	16.5	24.8	17.1
Silicone band methods	10.0	17.7	7.3
Spring clip	31.7	36.5	8.5
Hysteroscopy (Essure)	1.64	–	–
Vasectomy	11.3		No association

Source: Adapted from American College of Obstetricians and Gynecologists. Practice bulletin no. 133: Benefits and risks of sterilization. *Obstet Gynecol* 2013;121(2 Pt .1):392–404. PMID: 23344305 and Basinski (2010).

SELECTED READINGS

American College of Obstetricians and Gynecologists. Committee opinion no. 642: Increasing access to contraceptive implants and intrauterine devices to reduce unintended pregnancy. *Obstet Gynecol* 2015;126(4):e44–e48. PMID: 26393458

American College of Obstetricians and Gynecologists. Committee opinion no. 670: Immediate postpartum long-acting reversible contraception. *Obstet Gynecol* 2016;128(2):e32–e37. PMID: 27454734

American College of Obstetricians and Gynecologists. Committee opinion no. 672: Clinical challenges of long-acting reversible contraceptive methods. *Obstet Gynecol* 2016;128(3):e69–e77. PMID: 27548557

American College of Obstetricians and Gynecologists. Practice bulletin no. 186: Long-acting reversible contraception: implants and intrauterine devices. *Obstet Gynecol* 2017;130(5):e251–e269. PMID: 29064972

Damm P, Mathiesen ER, Petersen KR, Kjos S. Contraception after GDM. *Diabetes Care* 2007;30(Suppl. 2):S200–S205

Grigoryan OG, Grodnitskaya EE, Andreeva EN, Shestakova MV, Melnichenko GA, Dedov II. Contraception in perimenopausal women with diabetes mellitus. *Contraception* 2006;22:198–206

REFERENCES

American College of Obstetricians and Gynecologists. Practice bulletin no. 133: Benefits and risks of sterilization. *Obstet Gynecol* 2013;121(2 Pt .1):392–404. PMID: 23344305

American College of Obstetricians and Gynecologists. Committee opinion no. 620: Salpingectomy for ovarian cancer prevention. *Obstet Gynecol* 2015;125(1): 279–281. PMID: 25560145

Banks E, Berrington A, Casabonne D. Overview of the relationship between use of progestogen-only contraceptives and bone mineral density. *BJOG* 2001; 108(12):1214–1221. PMID: 11843382

Basinski CM. A review of clinical data for currently approved hysteroscopic sterilization procedures. *Rev Obstet Gynecol* 2010;3(3):101–110. PMID: 21364861

Branum AM, Jones J. Trends in long-acting reversible contraception use among U.S. women aged 15–44. NCHS data brief, no 188. Hyattsville, MD, National Center for Health Statistics, 2015. PMID: 25714042

Danis RB, Della Badia CR, Richard SD. Postpartum permanent sterilization: could bilateral salpingectomy replace bilateral tubal ligation? *J Minim Invasive Gynecol* 2016;23(6):928–932. PMID: 27234430

Deslypere JP, Thiery N, Vermeulen A. Effect of long-term hormonal contraception in plasma lipids. *Contraception* 1985;31:633–642. PMID: 4042661

Godsland IF, Crook D, Simpson R, et al. The effects of different formulations of oral contraceptive agents on lipid and carbohydrate metabolism. *N Engl J Med* 1990;323:1375–1381. PMID: 2146499

Goldstuck ND, Steyn PS. The intrauterine device in women with diabetes mellitus type I and II: a systematic review. *ISRN Obstet Gynecol* 2013:814062. PMID: 24396605

Greene MF. Prevention and diagnosis of congenital anomalies in diabetic pregnancy. *Clin Perinatol* 1993;20:533–547. PMID: 8222466

Grigoryan OG, Grodnitskaya EE, Andreeva EN, Chebotnikova TV, Melnichenko GA. Use of the NuvaRing hormone-releasing system in late reproductive-age women with type 2 diabetes mellitus. *Gynecol Endocrinol* 2008;24:99–104. PMID: 2146499

Kim C, Siscovick DS, Sidney S, Lewis CE, Kiefe CI, Koepsell TD. Oral contraceptive use and association with glucose, insulin, and diabetes in young adult women: the CARDIA study. *Diabetes Care* 2002;25(6):1027–1032. PMID: 12032110

Kjos SL, Peters RK, Xiang A, Thomas D, Schaefer U, Buchanan TA. Contraception and the risk of type 2 diabetes mellitus in Latina women with prior gestational diabetes mellitus. *JAMA* 1998;280:533–538. PMID: 9707143

Kjos SL, Shoupe D, Douyan S, et al. Effect of low-dose oral contraceptives on carbohydrate and lipid metabolism in women with recent gestational diabetes: results of a controlled, randomized, prospective study. *Am J Obstet Gynecol* 1990;163:1822–1827. PMID: 2256489

Liew DFM, Ng CSA, Yong YM, et al. Long term effects of Depo-Provera on carbohydrate and lipid metabolism. *Contraception* 1985;31:51–64. PMID: 3157546

Lopez LM, Grimes DA, Schulz KF. Steroidal contraceptives: effect on carbohydrate metabolism in women without diabetes mellitus. *Cochrane Database Syst Rev* 2014;4:CD006133. PMID: 24788670

Meade TW. Oral contraceptives, clotting factors and thrombosis. *Am J Obstet Gynecol* 1982;142(6 Pt. 2):758–761. PMID: 6801980

Miller E, Hare JW, Cloherty JP, Dunn PH, Gleason RE, Soeldner JS, Kitzmiller JL. Elevated maternal hemoglobin A1c in early pregnancy and major congenital anomalies in infants of diabetic mothers. *N Engl J Med* 1981;304:1331–1334. PMID: 7012627

Pal N, Broaddus RR, Urbauer DL, Balakrishnan N, Milbourne A, Schmeler KM, Meyer LA, Soliman PT, Lu KH, Ramirez PT, Ramondetta L, Bodurka DC, Westin SN. Treatment of low-risk endometrial cancer and complex atypical hyperplasia with the levonorgestrel-releasing intrauterine device. *Obstet Gynecol* 2018;131(1):109–116. PMID: 29215513

Shinar S, Blecher Y, Alpern S, Many A, Ashwal E, Amikam U, Cohen A. Total bilateral salpingectomy versus partial bilateral salpingectomy for permanent sterilization during cesarean delivery. *Arch Gynecol Obstet* 2017;295(5):1185–1189. PMID: 28285425

Skouby SO, Anderson O, Saurbrey N, et al. Oral contraception and insulin sensitivity: in vivo assessment in normal women and women with previous gestational diabetes. *J Clin Endocrinol Metab* 1987;64:519–523. PMID: 3102539

Skouby SO, Kuhl C, Molsted-Pedersen L, et al. Triphasic oral contraception: metabolic effects in normal women and those with previous gestational diabetes. *Am J Obstet Gynecol* 1985;153:495–500. PMID: 3933351

Speroff L, DeCherney A. Evaluation of a new generation of oral contraceptives. The Advisory Board of the New Progestins. *Obstet Gynecol* 1993;81:1034–1047. PMID: 8497347

Trussell J. Contraceptive efficacy. In *Contraceptive Technology*. 20th ed. Hatcher RA, Ed. New York, NY, Ardent Media, 2011

U.S. Medical Eligibility Criteria for Contraceptive Use, 2010. *Morbid Mortal Wkly Rep* 2010;59:1–86. PMID: 20559203

Vicente L, Mendonca D, Dingle M, Duarte R, Boavida JM. Etonogestrel implant in women with diabetes mellitus. *Europ J Contracep Repro Health Care* 2008;13:387–395. PMID: 19117254

Wilson ES, Cruickshank J, McMaster M, et al. A prospective controlled study of the effect on blood pressure of contraceptive preparations containing different types of dosages and progestogen. *Br J Obstet Gynaecol* 1984;91:1254–1260. PMID: 6440589

Xiang AH, Kawakubo M, Kjos SL, Buchanan TA. Long-acting injectable progestin contraception and risk of type 2 diabetes in Latino women with prior gestational diabetes mellitus. *Diabetes Care* 2006;29:613–617. PMID: 16505515

Index

CPSIA information can be obtained
at www.ICGtesting.com
Printed in the USA
FFHW012216200619
53121100-58776FF